Vile Jelly

One Man's Journey with Medicines, Glaucoma and Cataracts

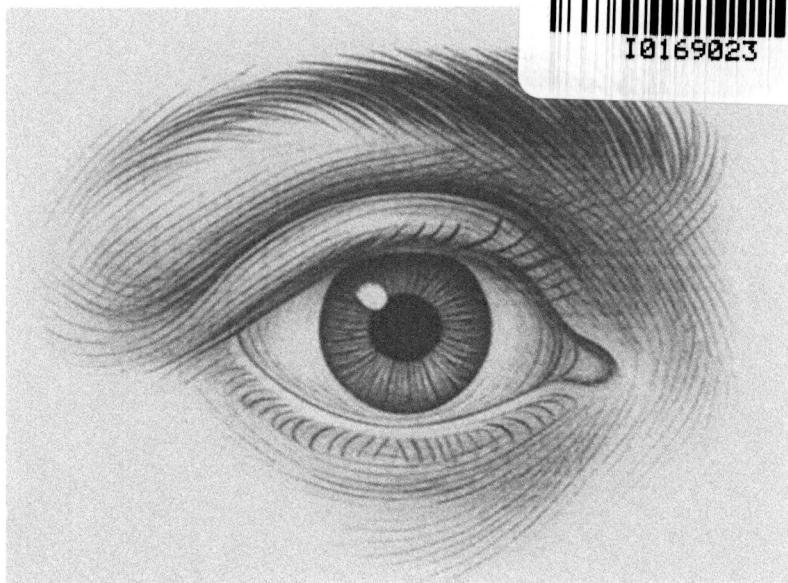

Dr Adrian Jarvis

Vile Jelly: One Man's Journey with Medicines, Glaucoma and Cataracts

Other books by Dr Adrian Jarvis

Chasing Shadows: The Search for Rod Evans
Sculpting In Rock: Deep Purple 1968-70
Infinite and Beyond: Deep Purple 1993-2022
The Aviator: The Life and Music of Steve Morse

Cover design by Guy D. Corp—www.grafixCORP.com

STAIRWAY≡PRESS

STAIRWAY PRESS—APACHE JUNCTION

www.stairwaypress.com
1000 West Apache Trail, Suite 126
Apache Junction, AZ 85120 USA

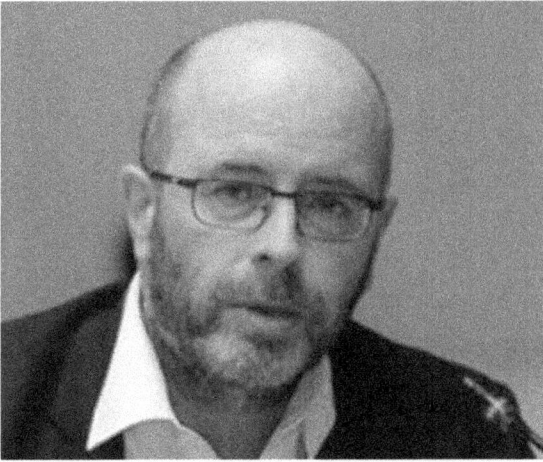

About the Author

DR ADRIAN JARVIS is a lecturer and educator at University of Huddersfield. Beyond the classroom, he has penned several books on rock music, including *Chasing Shadows: The Search for Rod Evans*, a compelling investigation into the elusive early Deep Purple vocalist; *Sculpting in Rock: Deep Purple 1968-70*, a detailed chronicle of the band's formative years; *Infinite and Beyond: Deep Purple 1993-2022*, an extensive look at their later evolution; and *The Aviator: The Life and Music of Steve Morse*, a tribute to the legendary guitarist.

With *Vile Jelly: One Man's Journey with Medicines, Glaucoma and Cataracts*, Dr Jarvis brings his meticulous research and personal narrative skills to the realm of medical experience, offering a unique and poignant perspective on his personal health journey.

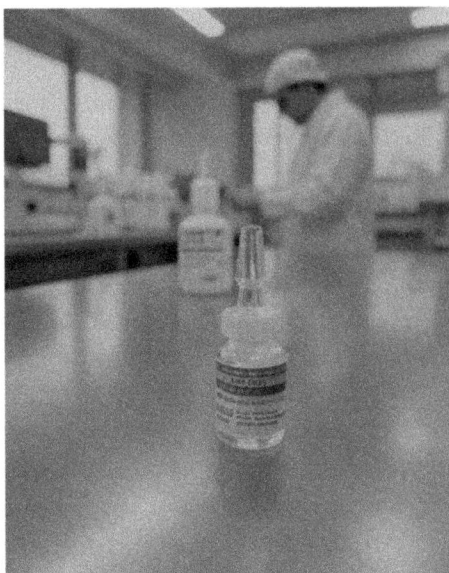

Prologue: The Panic in Sainsbury's Car Park

BAD NEWS IS often a case of asymmetries. It can be delivered at a banal location, such as the in-store pharmacy at a supermarket in the town of Huddersfield at which I was standing with Karen. It can also be devastating for the recipient—me—but a matter of supreme indifference to the deliverer—the pharmacist, or, anyway, the woman staffing the place.

The bad news in question?

'We're not going to be able to get the brimonidine tartrate with timolol.'

'What? Not at all?' I asked, incredulous.

'No,' she confirmed, 'I've contacted the supplier and they are listing it as out-of-stock.'

'When will it be in stock?'

'I don't know. Could be weeks or months. I just don't know.'

'Weeks or months!' I spluttered, 'But I need it now!'

I looked at Karen for moral support. She was always ready to give it, but, like the woman behind the counter, she did not really understand what the missing medicine meant to me.

Of the three eye drops that I was compelled to take twice a day, it was the only one that I had used up completely. The other two were not yet exhausted: I still had a small amount left—enough to last a day or two—and, anyway, the pharmacy had those 'in stock'. But the Brimonidine tartrate with timolol? Gone! I had anticipated some days earlier that it might need ordering in—that was standard—and had put in my prescription request in good time. But I did not imagine that it would not be obtainable at all.

If I did not get it, I would go blind. It was that simple. Not immediately. But the clock that it was supposed to pause would resume its remorseless countdown... I did not want to think about it.

I could feel my cheeks flushing and my body temperature rising.

Was this, I wondered, what it was like to go cold turkey?

'What if it was something I needed or I was going to die?' I asked— not rhetorically.

The woman behind the counter merely shrugged.

'Oh, so I would just have to die, then,' I said with bitter sarcasm.

'That's not what I meant, sir,' she said, barely concealing her annoyance.

This was getting nowhere. There was no alternative but just to be positive.

'So what can I do?'

The woman seemed relieved that I was not going along the 'difficult customer' route and responded accordingly.

'You can contact your GP and ask them to put the prescription back on the spine, where it can be accessed by other pharmacists. You can see if any of them have got the stuff.'

The 'spine' was an online platform listing outstanding prescriptions that could be accessed by any pharmacy. Only one pharmacy at a time could process any prescriptions displayed on it. This was shortly to become important.

'But,' I drew the conclusion, 'You're saying it's the supplier. Presumably, none of the other pharmacies will have it either.'

'Honestly, sir,' the woman behind the counter sympathized, 'It's like we're living in the Third World.'

'Well,' I said, 'I've just spent a lot of time in two Third World countries where I could have bought the drops off the shelf at any pharmacy.'

This was not strictly true. The part about buying it off the shelf was, but the countries had been Malaysia and the United Arab Emirates, neither of which is exactly Third World. But I had made my point. She had also made hers, which was to hint at the severe problems being faced by Britain's National Health Service, the NHS, in general. She was probably blaming Brexit, which, by this stage, was taking on the properties of Emmanuel Goldberg in *1984*—a convenient scapegoat for everything that went wrong, whatever the circumstances. In fact, recent global supply chain issues and their ultimate cause, the COVID-19 pandemic, were just as likely culprits. Or, it could just have been good old fashioned British inefficiency. Malaysia and Dubai, with their quick and easy solutions to every problem, seemed further away than could be measured in miles.

Still, discussions of current affairs were not going to get me any eye drops. It was twenty to five in the afternoon. My GP closed at six. Plenty of time to get the prescription re-assigned. I called. I got through and the prescription was put back on to the spine. Now all I had to do was find a pharmacist that had some of the eye drops in stock. Thank God for smartphones. Both Karen and I, hanging around in the supermarket's fruit and vegetable section, got to work looking for local pharmacies on the internet. We both found ourselves staring at the usual Google-sorted list. There seemed to be quite a few options, but I had assumed that they would all be open until late. Most were going to close at five thirty or six o'clock. There was now an added time pressure.

'Here's one,' I said, picking the first on the list, 'I'll try that.'

I called. A wait. A guy answered. He said that he would check to see if he had any of the drops. More waiting. He came back. Sorry—he didn't have it and it was listed as out-of-stock by the supplier. I could feel my panic rising, like that of King Lear—*hysterica passio*!

I cut to the chase.

'Is this going to happen with every pharmacy?'

'We've all had some supply problems, for sure,' the guy at the end of the line told me, 'But you might find a pharmacy that just happens to have some in.'

'It's not very likely, is it? This is not like aspirin! Who's going to have a bottle on their shelves?'

'It's worth a try,' he said.

It had to be. I rang off. Quarter past five. I tried the next pharmacy on the list.

Have you got the stuff? I asked the guy who answered. Yes, he confirmed. Yes! I was suddenly happy again. He took the prescription off the spine.

'We should be able to go and get it tonight,' I said to Karen.

Sorry, the guy said. It's the wrong formulation. It does not include the timolol. Deflated. Disappointed. Can you get the correct stuff? He checked. Out of stock; not sure when it's coming in. He said that he would return the prescription to the spine.

Karen and I walked back to the car in a sullen silence. It was a drizzly, chilly February day. Sitting in the passenger seat, I stared out through the windscreen, brooding.

'What do you want to do?' Karen asked.

I was mentally calculating. I had run out of the eye drops the previous evening but, even then, I had not had a full dose. The little plastic bottle had been so close to its last gasp that squeezing it into my eyes had produced little more than a puff of air and a few ineffectual bubbles of the precious liquid. I kidded myself that it had done some good. Obviously, I missed the dose that morning altogether and was increasingly in danger of missing the one due that evening. And there seemed no chance of getting the stuff before the sun rose the following morning with its demand for another dose. Damn my eyes! They were like medicine junkies! They stood to miss three—realistically, four— doses and that would be if I could secure a supply for the following evening. If I couldn't, who knew when I would be back to my full regimen? Until then, the pressures in my eyes would increase, crushing the sight out of my beleaguered optic nerves.

It had gone half past five. I took a final roll of the dice. I called one of the pharmacies that I had not so far tried.

'Hello,' I said, 'I wonder of you are able to get my prescription—it's on the spine.'

'Sure, I'll have a look,' the man at the other end of the phone said, having taken my identifying details. He saw the name of the eye drops and said that he would check. I was put on to an anxious hold. He came back:

'Yes, we can get that.'

'Really?' I said, flushed, lightened and refreshed by relief.

'Yes, we can get it in for tomorrow evening.'

'Oh, thank God!'

'Ah, hang on a minute,' he sounded preoccupied; for me, the panic was returning, 'It says here that the prescription is still with—' he named the previous pharmacy.

'Oh God,' I sighed, 'It should come off any second now. The guy there told me that he was putting it back on to the spine. I can give him a call.'

'If you could. I can't order it until it is back there.'

'Okay. Thank you. Thank you for your help.'

I rang off.

Thus is the life of anyone dependent on medicine—or a heroin addict for that matter. We have no choice. We are at the mercy of chemicals that our bodies need: if those chemicals are not forthcoming, our bodies become extremely hostile and stop doing the things that they are supposed to do. The problem in my case was that the heroes of my story, or anti-heroes might be more apt, were my eyes. No one wants to be ill, but I would guess that, given the choice, the majority of people would settle for having to take high blood pressure pills over fighting a daily battle against the gathering darkness of blindness.

I got the drops the next evening, but, by then, I had missed four doses. I could only guess at the damage done to my eyes. Perhaps none, but did I really want to take that bet? The longer the suppliers took, the more I lost. And what was lost could never be recovered. The best that I could hope for was a cessation, a stabilisation, a reprieve.

It is no accident that blindness is a big theme of literature. I would be staggered to be told that no PhD theses on the subject grace the shelves of the world's university libraries. One iconic blind character is Tiresias, the sightless prophet from Sophocles, who, in a more recent incarnation, is the 'old man with wrinkled dugs' through whose head runs the stream of consciousness that is T. S. Eliot's *The Waste Land*. The loss of his physical sight is compensated for by the gift of insight and foreknowledge. Not so Pozzo, from Beckett's *Waiting for Godot*, who mysteriously loses his vision between the play's acts. For him physical blindness is a symbol of his deeper lack of vision, not to mention the brutal grind of 'accursed time'.

Then there is the most horrific of all, Gloucester from *King Lear*, who, for the most minor of transgressions, has his eyes graphically plucked out and stamped on, his tormentor, Cornwall, intoning, 'out, vile jelly' as he goes about his grisly work. *Lear* is very much about seeing—seeing physically, seeing morally and seeing metaphorically.

As, the evening after the panic in Sainsbury's car park, I finally got around to squirting a cooling drop of brimonidine tartrate with timolol into each of my eyes, I was solely concerned with the first entry on that list.

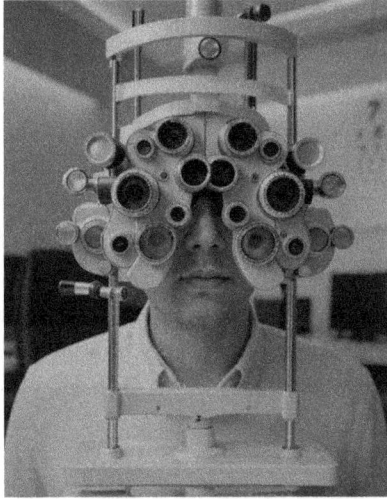

Chapter 1—Severely Damaged Eyes

'WHAT'S THAT ON the stage, mate?' Santosh, who was always known simply as 'Tosh', asked, 'Flowers, or something like that?'

We were standing at the back of the school hall. The end-of-the-year assembly was shortly to take place. The previous day had been spent with everyone—pupils, staff, the lot—taking part in a series of extra-curricular activities in the name of 'soft skills' building. One had involved creating life size figures using only newspapers and gaffer tape.

The results had been surprisingly impressive, comprising musicians playing double basses, young women checking their phones, businessmen carrying briefcases—a whole community of paper beings. They had been placed around the stage to showcase the day's outputs and to lend to this last gathering a suitably light-hearted tone. Tosh and I were no more than ten metres or so from the arrangement, but he was still unable to see it clearly. It was one of the moments—the quite rare moments—when the full extent of his visual impairment was revealed to me. He was not blind, but he was very close to it. At that moment, I could hardly imagine what the world looked like to him. I could not imagine full blindness at all.

Vile Jelly

In saying this, I am not being callous, because blindness is not all that easy to imagine. We tend to think of it in terms of Milton's 'darkness visible', as 'seen' dark. How do you conceive of the absence of a sense? Were our vision to disappear, our eyes, we somehow feel, would still work—they would just have nothing to look at. It is a bit like trying to put yourself mentally into the position of a dead person: you always seem to picture yourself experiencing death (if you don't believe me, try it). It is impossible to bring to mind a state of non-existence in which your past, present and future are gone: the first might as well have never happened, the second is not happening and the third never will. Gone. Voided. So it is with blindness. It is not seeing darkness; it is having no means of seeing anything.

Like death, it is something that you cannot believe will ever happen to you. At least, that is how I took it. Even when, years after that chat in the assembly hall, Tosh, who knew much more about the subject than I ever would, was advising me on how to get ready for it, I could not readily accept it. The senses are how we connect our minds, our inner lives, to the world.

Without them, what would we be? Disengaged entities.

People like Tosh, who have partial vision, are, in some ways, in a particularly misunderstood position. With someone who is completely blind, others know what they are dealing with, but that is not the case for those with some, but very little, vision. Tosh once related to me a story from his distant past in which he had been standing at a bus stop, nose pressed against the timetable in an attempt to discover when the next bus was due, only for a (less than cordial) guy walking past to shout, 'Are you fucking blind, or what?' Fortunately, what Tosh lacks in sight, he more than makes up for in sarcasm and he quickly riposted, 'Yeah, about 82%.'

I got to know Tosh because we both worked at an independent school in Cambridgeshire. I was Head of English, he was Head of German. We initially bonded not over vision but swearing. His first morning at work was a training day at the end of a Christmas holiday. He was sitting in the staff room paralysed by the usual nervousness that anyone in that position experiences; I had already been at the school for some years. I entered the room in medias res with another member of staff. I was not in a great mood.

'Who's fucking idea was it to get us in at this time?' I expostulated, 'I mean, for fuck's sake, day one after a long holiday! We could start this bullshit at ten. Why am I here at fucking eight thirty?'

Tosh later told me that he had been afraid that everyone at a school like that would be stuffy and correct (he had previously been used to the laidback atmosphere of a state-run college); my swearing reassured him that he might find a niche after all.

He told me that he had studied at St John's College Cambridge. When I told him that I had been at Keble College Oxford, he mistakenly believed that to be where I got my post-graduate qualifications. It took a while to convince him that I had been there as an undergraduate. Perhaps I did not come across as a typical 'Oxford Man'. Tosh was certainly an unlikely Cantabrian. Short, northern and a heavy smoker, he was proof that Oxbridge is a broader church than is often appreciated: we both were. By amazing coincidence, he had known my sister twenty years earlier when they had been on the same training course for the 'year abroad' that they would take during their modern languages degrees.

I am not sure when Tosh and I first discussed our eyes. I am not, for that matter, sure that it was ever brought up explicitly. Perhaps the closest to an opening conversation on the topic was when I spotted him sitting at a huge computer monitor that had been placed in the staff work room for his use and as was his custom, he had enlarged the text to 150%.

'Bloody Hell, mate,' I said, a little—in retrospect—insensitively, 'Why have you got that so large?'

'Er, so I can fucking read it!' was the characteristic response.

A similar relationship between Tosh and computer screens was apparent on the occasion that he came around to my place to watch a soccer World Cup clash between England and Uruguay. He missed a lot of the detail, the fact that he sat with his face millimeters from the screen notwithstanding. By his own admission, he has never been great at calling offsides. The next day, a pupil asked me where I had watched the game; upon reporting that I had watched it with 'Mr Ghosh', a girl in the class remarked that this was, 'So sweet!' Presumably, this came from a belief on her part that teachers are not supposed to be living normal lives and anything they do that smacks of one is to be treated with glaring condescension. Or maybe it had more to do with the way that those suffering adverse physical conditions tend to be framed by others—a word I use advisedly.

Susan Sontag has written about this, exploring how various illnesses have metaphorical connotations attached to them. She analysed tuberculosis, cancer and AIDS, but blindness, too, is frequently freighted with deeper meanings. The list of literary instances given in the previous chapter hint at the two main tropes—the wise blind person and non-literal blindness. The blind are often shown as possessing levels of perception and insight denied to those with all their senses: Tiresias is merely one example. Why this should be is perhaps a function of what is to such characters the physical world's lack of presence. Because of this, the notion runs, blind people spend their time thinking deeply about existence. Hence, they are able to dispense sage pieces of advice to their sighted peers, the implication being that sight is, in some way, the disability and blindness the blessing.

The second metaphor is all about emotional and spiritual states. When Ian Gillian of my favorite rock band Deep Purple sings, 'I'm a blindman and my world is pale', he is not claiming to be physically blind. He is saying that he is down, depressed, lonely perhaps. These are only some of the states associated with being figuratively blind: naïve, easily hoodwinked, foolish are also covered, as are many others. They all add to the pattern of meanings that are woven into the dramatic tapestry of *King Lear* and its like. In short, being blind is not just being blind: it implies a whole condition of life that separates the person so afflicted from their environment.

Such thoughts preoccupied me as I sat in a hospital room in Huddersfield talking to a female consultant who was taking me through the eye scan to which I had just been subjected. This was about seven years after the conversation with Tosh in the school hall. By now, my situation was not so different from his.

'Your glaucoma is very advanced,' the consultant said, pointing to a picture on her computer screen that looked like a negative of a distant galaxy.

'If you look here,' she went on, 'you can see that most of the optic nerve is in the red in your left eye. There is a little in the white, but not very much.'

I could not really see that, to be honest. For a start, the picture was not very clear, but between glaucoma and the huge cataract that had developed in my right eye, my capacity for picking up visual information was not at its best.

'Any intervention would not be without risk,' she concluded.

She measured my pressures, which meant resting my chin on a brace as a large machine shone a laser-like light into my eyes.

'Mmm,' she said, 'Eighteen and nineteen.'

Eighteen in my right eye, nineteen in my left. This was a slight source of hope. I had always been led to believe that the magic number was twenty. Anything above it was the danger zone, anything below was okay. This reading was not all that promising but I was in that room in the first place because my most recent reading—three months earlier—had returned nineteen and twenty-three. My cheer was not to last long.

'I'm going to dilate your irises,' she said.

I nodded. She put some gunk in my eyes and sent me to sit in the waiting room for fifteen minutes or so.

This was my first chance to reflect on what was going on.

That was that my eyes seemed to have made a deal with each other to ruin my life. To put this in more medical language, I was suffering, as the consultant had said, from glaucoma, and had been for some thirteen years. In case you are unaware of what glaucoma is, it is a disease in which the eyes' pressures are consistently too high.

'Eye pressure' refers to the amount of aqueous humour inside the eyeball. Of this, there is an optimum and, providing that the optimum is more-or-less maintained, the eye will work perfectly well—with the proviso that it is still prone to myopia, macular degeneration and any number of other ailments. For anyone interested enough, the relationships between the different substances inside the eyeball can be measured by use of Goldman's Equation, that is:

$$P^o = \frac{F - U}{C} + P_v$$

Where P^o is the intraocular pressure in millimeters of mercury, F is the rate of aqueous humour formation in microliters per minute, U is the resorption of aqueous humour through the uveoscleral route, C is the facility of outflow in microliters per minute per millimeter of mercury and Pv is the episcleral venous pressure in millimeters of mercury.

Got that?

What this means is that if the eye contains too much aqueous humour, very bad things result. Most alarmingly, the optic nerve is damaged. Without an optic nerve, it is impossible to see. People who are fully blind can have nothing wrong with their eyes per se; their eyes can be beautiful, models of everything an eye can be, but they are not connected to the brain via the optic nerve. It is a bit like having a desktop CPU and a monitor, but no cable with which to attach one to the other. Left untreated, then, glaucoma is the path of progressive blindness. The quantity of aqueous humour is expressed in terms of a pressure number. Broadly, the lower that number is, the better. Somewhere around twelve is considered good. Fifteen or sixteen is acceptable. Much higher than that and alarm bells start to ring.

Glaucoma cannot be cured. And, as I have already said, whatever sight is destroyed by its ravages is gone forever. Typically, glaucoma results in the loss of peripheral vision. The visual 'fields' close in, restricting sight to an ever-smaller dot in the centre until pfft, only darkness remains. Fortunately, it can be treated and managed. There are various ways in which this can be done, but by far the most common is eye drops. These oblige the sufferer to squirt into their eyes a cocktail of medicines—determined by the severity of their case—a couple of times a day. Operations are possible, but tend to be used as a last resort, which was why the consultant's talk of *interventions* represented a considerable escalation.

I was called back into her room.

'Twenty three and twenty six,' she told me matter-of-factly.

'That's not so good,' I said, trying to match her tone, but barely managing to conceal my disappointment.

She returned to the photographs of my optic nerves.

'Have you had some sort of head trauma?' she asked.

I was a little taken aback.

'Well, if I did, it didn't stop me getting a PhD, so more of that, please!'

'Seriously,' she said. 'Your left eye is considerably worse than your right. That is strange. Glaucoma is usually more symmetrical. I think I'm going to send you for an MRI scan.'

'What?' I said, now genuinely worried.

'Don't worry,' she reassured me. 'It's more to rule things out than anything else.'

When I rejoined the remarkably patient Karen in the waiting room, it was to deliver the kind of news that did not normally accompany such moments. For a start, I had a new prescription. I was now on tablets that I was required to take four times a day. Alongside the three lots of eye drops. Then there was the little matter of the scan...

We walked to the hospital's pharmacy and, upon learning that it would take a while for my prescription to be curated, we sat in the adjacent café—with a coffee for me and a fruit tea for Karen.

'How do you feel?' Karen asked.

What could I say?

The truthful answer was *shocked*. I had been a diligent user of eye drops ever since they had first been prescribed for me. I would have struggled to identify even one occasion on which I had failed to take them. There must have been some in thirteen years, for sure, but they were so few that they had long since become buried in the murk of forgetfulness.

It was easy to feel cheated. I had done my bit. Attended every appointment. Done everything I had been told to do. Listened to every scrap of advice. But I had still reached this place! How was that fair? Then again, what was that place? My vision was not great, it was true, but that was largely because of the cataract, which the consultant had told me was operable. Otherwise…well, I could see out of my troublesome left eye. Probably nowhere near as well as I had been able to in the past. If a comparison had been possible, I would no doubt have been appalled at what it revealed. But that was simply not going to happen and what I had was an eye that seemed to work okay. It didn't hurt. I didn't notice that it was getting worse. That is probably the most pernicious aspect of glaucoma: you don't know that you've got it. At least, there is no sign that you can personally recognise. In my more darkly satirical moments, I have even wondered whether it exists at all; after all, I only take the drops because someone tells me to, but what if, for some nefarious reason beyond my ken, they are lying? What if the whole thing is just a conspiracy? Abraham Lincoln famously said that you can't fool all of the people all of the time, but—here's the rub—how would we ever know?

In answer to Karen's question, I simply said:

'It is what it is, isn't it? There's nothing I can do about it.'

'You've had an MRI scan before, haven't you?' she asked.

I had. About fifteen years earlier in a bookshop in the picturesque Cambridgeshire city of Ely, I had suffered a seizure. I know this sounds like a scene from a BBC drama that might have been made in the mid-1980s, but it really did happen. I had been walking through the town and suddenly came over all—well, what? *Weird* would be putting it mildly. In the bookshop, I sat at a low table in the children's section, 'just for a minute'. The next thing I knew I was lying on my back with a paramedic crouched over me applying an oxygen mask to my face and saying my name. Every muscle in my body ached and my tongue, which I had presumably been biting, felt like it had been hacked at with a knife. Most awful of all was the fact that I could remember nothing. Actually, that is not quite true. I could remember that there was an onion factory in the nearby town of Chatteris. Apart from that, it was as though my entire personality had drained away.

Fortunately, Sally, my girlfriend at that time, was with me and she was—like Karen—one of the many massively resourceful women with whom I have been lucky to be surrounded over the years. She had summoned an ambulance and hauled me into the recovery position, helped by a shop assistant. She then accompanied me to Addenbrookes

Hospital in Cambridge and provided me with transport in the other direction, putting up my very confused self at her place. Over the next few hours, I began to recover my cognitive functions, although I am sure that my memory has not been quite what it had been ever since. The following day, I went back to the hospital to meet with a consultant.

'Do you know what it could be?' I asked him.

'Oh, it could be all kind of nasty things,' he told me, jovially.

'Oh,' I said, not quite seeing the humour in the situation.

'I wouldn't worry,' he said, 'You're probably epileptic, that's all.'

Phew, I thought, only epilepsy! Nothing too serious then...

It was not epilepsy. I never found out what it was. In my more fanciful moments, I have wondered whether the glaucoma had its origins in that seizure, but my rational self knows that things do not work that way.

'This might put a few things that we've been planning off, or back,' I said to Karen in the hospital coffee shop, pensively sipping my Americano.

She accepted what I was saying with characteristic stoicism. We had not been in Huddersfield for long—having come back from living in Dubai—but we harboured plans to go abroad again, a decision that was rendered easy by my only having a temporary contract. Since I was already well over halfway through it, I was beginning to think about the next step. Or, rather, I had been. Suddenly there were contexts I hadn't initially taken into account.

Karen just nodded.

'Get your eyes sorted out and then we'll think about what we're going to do,' she said.

We picked up the prescription and it became a part of my regular routine: three lots of eye drops twice a day and a pill every six hours. The pills had a habit of starting to dissolve before I could take a sip of water, filling my mouth with nasty tasting powder. Still, they had the desired effect; at a follow-up appointment a couple of weeks later, I found out that my pressures were back down to safe levels. By then, I had run out of the tablets, but the cheery doctor (I never saw that consultant again) told me that he wouldn't prescribe any more because they were 'only a short term solution'. I wondered if this was tempting fate but kept my mouth shut.

As for the MRI scan, I heard nothing. Perhaps the consultant had forgotten about it or thought better of it. My mistake was to rely on the appointment being communicated by text.

The flat in which Karen and I were staying received its post to a box in a separate room. We were somewhat negligent as far as checking it was concerned. Most of our own communicating was done by email or social media, so the old-fashioned analogue approach was easy to forget about. By pure chance, we happened to open the door of the box and reach inside one Wednesday night, only to find a letter, sent nearly a fortnight earlier, informing me that I had an appointment for a scan two days hence. I wondered why the NHS was contacting me in such an archaic manner. After all, they had texts, emails and an app that they could have used, but there I was holding a scrappy sheet of paper, a sheet of paper that I had very nearly overlooked. I had complacently been telling myself that the scan was not going to happen. Now I knew that it was, the mouse teeth of worry started to gnaw at the edges of my imagination.

I Googled what the MRI scan might be intended to find. My advice would be never to do this. Five minutes with anything that even remotely resembles a medical textbook is enough to get even the most confident of people convinced that they are suffering from half the ailments in it. I once looked at a family health encyclopedia to rule out asthma as the cause of some wheezing that I was doing only to come away believing that I had not only asthma, but a collapsed lung, heart disease and diabetes. Tosh refuses to take a psychopathy test for much the same reason. On this occasion, my internet search returned the result that MRI scans for glaucoma would most often be checking for eye cancer, which is fatal if not quickly treated. I expressed my concern (read: uncontrollable panic) to Karen.

'The consultant would have said something if they were looking for cancer, wouldn't she?' I said, reaching for any available twig of reassurance.

'Yes,' Karen replied, 'I think they've got to.'

'They've got to be up front.'

'I think so.'

Karen was working on the day of the scan, so, alone, I took an Uber to the hospital, fidgeting in my seat as a growing sense of unease overtook me. When I arrived, I followed the directions in the letter to the scanner room, which was in a basement. That did not calm me down, but the mundanity of what I found did. Nothing was very high tech. There was hardly anyone around. I asked a passing nurse where I was supposed to go. She told me to put my coat in a locker and report to a waiting room—actually just a few chairs in a corridor—from where I would be called.

The atmosphere seemed at odds with the purpose of the place. Presumably, people with all manner of serious ailments passed through there on a regular basis, but nothing said 'danger', or 'warning', or 'be careful'. I could have been waiting for a haircut. Somewhere down a corridor, I heard a couple of women, employees I guessed, laughing. Surely, it was inconceivable that here—bland, unexciting, here—could be where I would hear any life-changing or earth-shattering news.

The technician who was due to perform the scan appeared from behind some double doors and instructed me to accompany her. In films, MRI scans always have something distinctly sci-fi about them. The patient lies down while a laser beam passes over him or her and an x-ray image of his or her head, clearly showing the brain, appears on a nearby screen. Real life—it turned out—is a little different. The scanner resembled a large sun bed and, while it was no doubt a piece of incredibly sophisticated technology, it did not especially appear to be. It looked a bit worn, a bit used, a bit industrial. I was instructed to lie down, the 'bed' being more comfortable than it looked. I was given some headphones. This I was not expecting, especially as they were pumping out a radio station specialising in '80s classics (*Always on My Mind* by Pet Shop Boys was playing when I put them on). I then had to rest my head on a support and was—there is no other way of putting it—clamped in. This was to ensure that my head didn't move around while it was being scanned. The procedure was far more than a light beam passing over the body; I was to be in there for around twenty minutes. A lid that was half a cylinder was closed over me. One last, 'everything okay?' from the technician and it began.

It was a weird experience, but a surprisingly relaxing one. Lights danced in front of my eyes. The headphones quickly became irrelevant because the machine was noisy. Extremely noisy. At times, it made a sound like a robot sobbing. At others, it whirred like a demented washing machine. At one point, it produced a bass beat like the synth opening of any number of the eighties songs to which I was being subjected: the technician later told me that one guy had asked if he could sample it for use in a piece of music. I began to feel a soporific wave wash over me. My lids became heavy, my head drowsy. I was conscious that falling asleep in there was probably not permitted and I did my best to fight against it.

I was kept awake by the jolt of the machine's cycle suddenly ending. No tapering effect, no preparatory beeps. It just stopped, midway through a song by Simple Minds. The technician lifted the lid and efficiently removed the brace from my neck.

'Okay?' I asked, my tone that of someone anticipating an instant result.

'You should hear something in a couple of weeks,' the technician said.

Adrian Jarvis

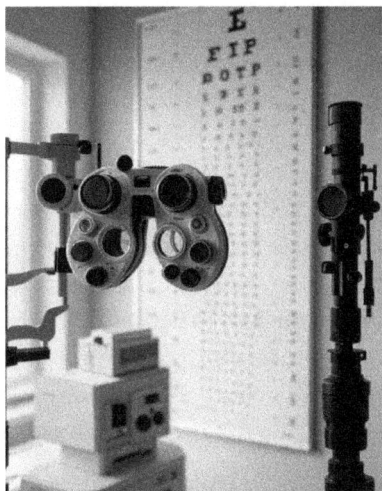

Chapter 2—Diagnosed

I DON'T REMEMBER ever going along the Kubler-Ross curve with glaucoma.

Originally devised as a way to explain the stages of grief, the curve has since been applied to any form of change, especially that of receiving a chronic medical diagnosis. The different emotions that a person feels during the period of re-adjustment are plotted on it, reaching a nadir, before moving upwards in a positive direction.

The first stage is denial: an afflicted, or affected, person will refuse to believe that the worst is true. That quickly gives way to anger when reality becomes impossible to ignore; the anger often takes the form of, 'Why me? Why not someone else?' After anger is bargaining, the more-or-less deluded attempt to come to some accommodation with the change, diagnosis, whatever. This might involve the person thinking, 'Okay, I've got this problem, but I can still do the things that I want', or 'It probably will not make much difference or get any worse.' The lowest point is reached with what comes next, depression. This follows from the apparent exhausting of all options and the final realisation of what is actually happening. At this point, though, the curve takes a radical upswing as the person achieves acceptance: they cease to fight and begin to find some sort of positives in their predicament.

I avoided all of this, partly, perhaps, because of the way in which the news of my glaucoma was delivered to me, and partly because of the impact that it had on my life. Interestingly, Tosh was given the news in 2019 that he was diabetic and also swerved the curve, so to speak. He confessed that he had been drinking Coke like it was going out of style for years, so, intellectually, had long accepted that something like diabetes was a no-brainer for him. That his newly discovered condition entailed the giving up of drinks such as cider was, if anything, a felicitous side effect as he 'couldn't stand the fucking stuff anyway.' Tosh's equivalent of Kubler-Ross's final stage is very nearly his personal mantra: 'It is what it is.'

As for my eyes, I was first alerted to the possibility that not all was right with them when I was having my annual vision test in the darkened consultation room of a high street optician. I had been through the reading of ever smaller letters on a screen and had tried to determine whether black lines were sharper against red or green backgrounds. To complete the examination, the optician performed a, purely routine, eye pressure test. I had done it many times before. It was no big deal. It had always ended with the optician giving me a cheery smile before swiftly moving on.

Not this time. He seemed troubled.

'Everything all right?' I asked.

'Mmmm,' he mumbled, preoccupied.

There was a pause. It was broken by him saying:

'I'm going to ask you to do a fields test.'

'Okay,' I said, still not spotting that we had now moved away from the everyday and towards the worrying.

I was taken into the room next door by one of the shop's assistants. It contained a chair in front of another large piece of machinery, one that, in various incarnations, was to become the bane of my life over the next decade or so. In front of the chair was a face rest and pad. Taking my place on the chair allowed me to look into a blank space with only a delicate lens between me and a single yellow light. In my hand was a clicker. The test was simple: I had to focus on the yellow light and click the clicker every time I saw a small green light anywhere else in the space. Some of the green lights were bright and appeared for as long as a second. Some were little more than pale pimples that flashed once and were gone. The test was taken one eye at a time.

I started with my right eye. A patch was placed over my left. A grinding noise accompanied the machine's operation. The test was simple enough. As far as I could tell, I could see everything that was thrown at me. At one point, a pre-recorded American woman's voice intoned, 'You're doing great!', to be followed shortly after by, 'Almost finished now.' Suddenly, the machine stopped.

'That's it,' the shop assistant said, 'Now for the left.'

The procedure was repeated. But it wasn't quite repeated. I was not clicking as often. I didn't see as many lights. Sometimes, I wasn't as sure that what I was seeing was a pale light and not just part of the general murk. The artificial American lady informed me that the test was over and I sat back. Somehow I knew that I had not done as well with my left eye, but I could not predict what that would mean.

I was taken back around to the original consultation room. The optician took the printouts of my test from the assistant.

'I suppose you flew through that, then,' he began, before glancing at what he had and stopping himself short, 'Oh!'

'Is there a problem?' I asked, disingenuously.

'You've got some field loss in your left eye,' he told me. 'That means that there are blind spots. Your eye pressures are also high. I'm reading twenty-seven and twenty-eight.'

'Is that bad?'

'I think that you should make an appointment with an eye specialist. Meanwhile, I will see you back here in a couple of weeks to fit your new glasses.'

I saw Sally that evening. We were heading to one of our favourite haunts for dinner, a hotel in the town of Huntingdon in Cambridgeshire that always managed to combine sophistication with a warm welcome and an excellent menu. We sat in some large comfortable armchairs in the lounge area with a low table in front of us on which rested the two glasses of Chardonnay from which we liberally sipped. I reported what had happened at the optician.

'What does high pressure mean?' she asked.

'Good question,' I replied, 'But, clearly, it is not a good thing.'

'It's probably something that can be treated and cured,' she said.

'Yes. Even so, I suppose that I had better go to see my doctor so that he can refer me to an eye specialist.'

'I'm sure that it's nothing much to worry about.'

I would not have called Sally a noted Pollyanna, but, on this occasion, I couldn't help feeling that she was being too optimistic.

'Has an optician ever given you that test where they blow air into your eye?' I asked her.

'Yes,' she said.

'But no-one's ever made too much of it?'

'No.'

I sipped my wine.

When I got around to meeting with him, my doctor was unimpressed. He argued that the loss of fields in my left eye could have had any number of causes and that my heightened pressures were likely to be a temporary thing. They were certainly not something about which I should be concerned. When I reported the conversation to the optician a couple of weeks later, he was horrified.

'I urge you to get a second opinion,' he said, 'If you do nothing, you could lose your peripheral vision until you can only see a pin prick in the centre...'

He illustrated this by making a tiny hole with his thumb and forefinger.

'Could I—lose all of my sight, then?'

'Potentially, yes,' he said.

It was with a slightly sick feeling in my gut that I tried on the expensive designer frames that I was there to fit to my face. It is only looking back at those events with a remove of time that it occurs to me that the word 'glaucoma' was not used.

At that point, I was living in a rented house in the town of March, Cambridgeshire. There is not a lot to say about March. It had a very convenient railway station, which happened to be directly opposite my house, and that was about it. There were a couple of pubs, quite a nice curry house and, anomalously, a sort-of fine dining restaurant. There was not much else. But there was an eye clinic. Or rather, there was a surgery that ran an eye clinic every couple of weeks or so. The building was one of those places that at the time I would have called 'boring', but, in hindsight, seems like a little Eden of tranquility and order. It was to be found in a leafy suburban street which came off the road out of the town centre. When I first went, by appointment, the car park was nearly empty. The building's interior was uncrowded and quiet. I was directed to sit in a small waiting room. No one else was there. I was called through to see the eye surgeon.

I have tended to anonymise people in this account, but, in this case, it is because I genuinely cannot remember the guy's name. This is not for any negative reason. He was a very personable individual and somewhat eccentric. Immaculately dressed in a suit and tie, his shiny dome of cranial baldness was fringed with close cropped hair. He greeted me with an air of jocularity and bonhomie. He asked me a few questions about myself and how I came to be there. I told him about the optician, omitting the role played by my doctor. He made a few notes. Did I feel any pain in my eyes? No. Did I notice any loss of vision? No, beyond normal short-sightedness.

'Right, let's have a look at these eyes of yours, shall we?' he said.

I rested my chin on a device made up of probes and lenses. Yellow dye was dropped onto my eyes. Lights were shone into them. Air was puffed into them.

'Mmm,' he said.

It was not a satisfied 'mmm', or a quizzical 'mmm', or a I-might-need-to-think-about-this 'mmm'. It was a I-had-hoped-we-wouldn't-find-that 'mmm'. I could only sit there, letting destiny do its work. He enjoined me to sit back and moved the machine away.

'Well, your pressures are high,' he said.

I did not reply. I was waiting for the inevitable.

'I think you've got glaucoma,' he said.

'Okay,' I said neutrally.

It was as unexciting as that. I felt no devastation. No sense of unfairness. No awareness of how, in that one moment, my life changed forever. I suppose that it was because—from my perspective—there were no real symptoms. What did higher pressures in my eyes mean to me? I could still see! I felt no pain. It seemed to be, at worst, a minor problem.

'Can it be cured?' I asked.

'Oh, no,' he replied, 'I'm afraid not. It's a guest for life.'

'Well, is there any treatment, then?' I persisted.

'Eye drops,' he said, producing a squeezy bottle that was comically small. It was for a concoction called Travatan.

'Put one drop of this in both eyes once a day, preferably in the evening. Come back in two weeks so that we can see how things are going.'

'One drop?' I asked, 'That does not seem like much.'

'One, maybe two,' he said, 'Use it sparingly. You don't need much of it.'

I took the bottle.

'This is like an indefinite thing, isn't it?' I said.

'Oh, yes,' he said, 'Forever and ever and ever.'

'Great!' I said with bitter sarcasm.

He laughed.

'I wouldn't be too alarmed,' he said, 'Glaucoma is very treatable. My job is to make sure that you die with exactly the same vision that you've got now.'

'In that case,' I said, 'I will be happy to let you get on with your job.'

He chuckled again.

'Take it once a day,' he reminded me as I got up to leave.

Once a day, every day, sounded like quite a lot, but it did not hit me too hard. After all, I reasoned, I clean my teeth twice a day, so what's one more minor routine? I'll get used to it.

'I'll see you in a couple of weeks,' I said.

'We'll make an appointment for you,' he said.

I walked back out to my Toyota MR2, which waited for me in the car park. I sat in the driver's seat for a few minutes thinking over what had just happened. In some ways, it was bad. But everything was so— light touch. A tiny toy bottle of medicine. One drop a day. One drop! As major medical emergencies go, this could have been worse. And if this was as bad as it got…I allowed myself an ironic smile. Perhaps I had less to worry about than that optician had led me to believe. Now I thought about it, he had been rather excitable. This would be a breeze.

I started up the ignition. The engine growled into life. I turned into the deserted street and headed for home.

Taking the drops every evening proved to be more annoying than I had anticipated. It was not the actual act—although the drops did sting occasionally—it was trying to remember whether I had taken them at all. Constantly repeated activities tend to become forgettable: who hasn't worried about whether they have locked the front door when leaving the house? In a similar way, I would find myself sitting on the sofa, or driving, or sipping a drink, wracking my brains for recollections of myself squeezing the mini bottle of Travatan into my unwilling eyes. The problem was that the medicine's instructions expressly stated that missed applications were to be moved on from; putting another drop in was not advised.

I expressed these worries when I next saw the eye surgeon.

'I wouldn't worry,' he said, 'the half-life of Travatan is about thirty-six hours—we only say to put it in every evening so that people don't start to habitually neglect applications.'

This was sort of reassuring: it left around a twelve-hour gap when my eyes were not being treated. But only when I forgot to put the drops in—which may or may not have happened. I could not recall either way.

He checked my pressures.

'Nineteen,' he said of my left eye, 'eighteen' of my right.

'It worked!' I exclaimed, falsely believing that the glaucoma dragon had been slain and I could go back to my normal life.

'That won't do at all,' he muttered.

'It's not good, then?'

'No. It's not good. I was hoping that the drops would have brought things down a lot more than that.'

Vile Jelly

That may have been the moment at which the gravity of my situation hit home. I had naively assumed that putting in a drop of Travatan every evening would solve the problem. It clearly had not. Yes, the pressures were below twenty, but only just. They were still on the high side. I had not yet been introduced to the fact that pressures are far from a constant: they can go up and down within the course of a day. Persistently high pressures are the problem.

'What can I do?' I asked.

Another tiny plastic bottle appeared. This one was for a product called Azarga.

'Take this twice a day,' the doctor said as he handed the bottle to me.

'Twice a day?' I repeated, a little bleakly.

'Yes.'

I took the bottle and considered it, troubled.

'I have just submitted my PhD thesis,' I said.

'Well done!' the surgeon said in a way that did not convey congratulations.

'Many of the opportunities that I might get from that are likely to be abroad,' I explained, 'Would this prevent me from taking any of those up?'

'Oh no!' he told me, 'Those decisions should never be driven by glaucoma. You can get these medicines abroad—they don't cost much.'

I felt relieved, although I probably should not have done.

I went away a man on a slippery slope. In only a couple of weeks, the glaucoma's rate of advance had accelerated. I was not that old—early forties. In theory, the disease had years and years in which to work its mischief.

Where would it go from here?

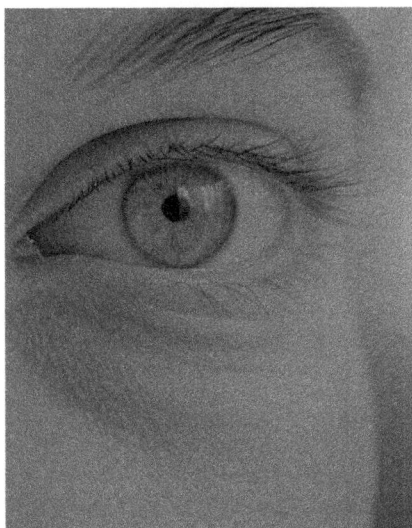

Chapter 3—Before and After

I THINK ABOUT glaucoma every day. Not all day. I can't say that. But a day does not go by on which I do not think about it in some way. Of course, I think about it every time I put in my eye drops—and the move to combine Travatan and Azarga was by no means the last time that my medication was adjusted. But the disease is on my mind at other times, too. It is a monkey on my back that just happens to be wielding the sword of Damocles while prepping a time bomb—because I know that, in all likelihood, I will eventually go blind.

The doctor in March may have constantly assured me that his job was to help me to die with exactly the same eyesight that I had when I first met him, but I never quite felt convinced. The speed with which my permanent eye drop regime had developed was scary and the pressures never stayed the same. They could be low one visit. Higher the next. My left eye was worse than my right. My left eye increasingly seemed to have a death wish. Which was ironic, because it had traditionally been the stronger of the two.

An optician I visited on one occasion told me that I was 'the unlucky one'. She was referring to my not having any of the pre-conditions that are usually present in glaucoma patients. I am not diabetic—the two things often go hand-in-hand. I am not of African, Asian or Hispanic descent. There is no history of glaucoma in my family (although given that most of my ancestors lived in extreme poverty and did not always reach a ripe old age, some of them could have had it without ever finding out). I was not over the age of fifty-five when I was diagnosed. I do not suffer from high blood pressure, migraines or any of the other ailments that can be risk factors. For me, the disease came out of nowhere. By rights, I should not have it. And yet, I do.

It has divided my life into two chapters. The first covers that of everything that happened pre-glaucoma. The second, post-glaucoma.

My pre-glaucoma life now seems like a time of prelapsarian innocence. My eyes have never been anyone's idea of perfect. In the sense of how they work, I mean. Short-sighted, then short- and long-sighted, they have been, at best, serviceable. To look at, as opposed to from, though, they have elicited many positive comments. They are not large, but they are blue; when not covered by the distorting lenses of glasses, they might even be called 'piercing'. I have always attributed that to my Irish ancestry. My father, from whom my English blood comes, had hazel eyes: I did not inherit my eye colour from him. My eyes were designed to overlook Celtic landscapes and raging northern seas. They are cold, like the climate that begat them.

But, if my eyes have any aesthetic qualities—I am not the best judge of that—they are as nothing next to my eyelashes, which have frequently been lauded, particularly by women, often with openly expressed envy. Girlfriends, friends, even my students, have all—usually with a gasp of surprise—told me how lovely they find my eyelashes. What can I say? Like most men, I can claim no expertise about what constitutes attractive eyelashes, so I usually take the compliments with an affectation of goofy modesty and move on.

That was the best part of the pre-glaucoma dispensation, the worst was in how I too often behaved. Anger. Envy. Sloth. Like anyone, I was an arrant committer of the seven deadly sins. I felt competitive with colleagues and friends. I worried about my work and did not always get the balance between urgent and important right. It all seems like arch foolishness now. What did it matter if I was a couple of days late giving back some marked work to the kids I taught? It made no difference to their final outcomes. What did it matter if I spent an annoyingly large amount on servicing my car? It was only money. Why did I argue about nonsense with my first wife, my girlfriends and casual acquaintances? I didn't care all that much about whatever we were arguing about: what did I think I might be gaining? Really? Nothing! Compared to a disease that could so easily turn into a disability, well, what did any of it matter?

I realise that this all sounds self-pitying. It is not. It reflects a newfound sense of realism. Glaucoma—probably any chronic degenerative disease—is a fact of life. It is not personal. You can be the nicest human being in the world. The most generous. Or, conversely, evil, cruel, fanatical. It is all the same to glaucoma. It does not give you a break. It does not censure. As far as it is concerned, a victim is a victim is a victim. You just have to accept it.

But it means that I now think according to the pre-and post-schema. I remember dinners with Sally, those trips to Marrakech and Vienna, that night in a Scottish hotel with Amanda—all belonged to the world before glaucoma. When I see the release dates for old films, I divide them into ones that were released pre-glaucoma and those that came out post-glaucoma. When I bring the past to mind, I ask of whatever I am recalling: 'did I have glaucoma then, or was that before I got it?' If it was afterwards, I try to remember where the eye drops fitted in—when did I take them? At what time of day? Were there any problems? When I consider the many years before glaucoma, it is a form of mental archaeology. I am looking at a buried civilization that always had the seeds of its own destruction within it. I should have been more alive to the possibility of something happening that would change everything forever.

Perhaps I was. As those pre-glaucoma days were coming to an end, I often found myself squinting at cinema screens through first my right eye, then my left. The difference between the brightness and sharpness of the right and the dullness of the left was stark. I just assumed that it was an aspect of the short-sightedness that has been my burden since the age of eleven. I now know that it was an as yet unnamed predator in the depths of my eyeballs, eating ravenously at my vision, stripping it bare, leaving nothing to the future.

Two people loomed large in the post-glaucoma world. The first was Karen. The other was Tosh. Through him, I met many other members of the unsighted and partially sighted community. I have often pondered the coincidence of my becoming involved with people suffering sight problems. It was not a plan by any means. Fate drew me in that direction.

As for Tosh, the most noticeable thing about him was how little he let his visual impairment bother him. Apart from a need to stare intensely at computer screens, there was not much about him to indicate that he only enjoyed 15% vision across both eyes. He was remarkably self-sufficient and positive. As my glaucoma grew steadily worse over the years, I took him as an inspiration.

He was, for example, quite the independent traveller. He was in the habit of taking what he called his 'northern tour' at least once every year. This was a rail trip around various places in Yorkshire and Lancashire to visit family and friends; Huddersfield was on the list of destinations. Even more impressively, he made lengthy visits every so often to Marburg in Germany, the town in which he had spent his undergraduate year abroad.

Only rarely did Tosh's visual impairment enter into my relationship with him. I would sit next to him at the back of the hall during school assemblies and quietly describe the contents of PowerPoint slides to him. I would sometimes read documents for him if the font was too small. Somewhat stereotypically, the weakness of his eyes was accompanied by the excellence of his ear: he was a superb singer. At his suggestion, we joined a barbershop group. We had a ball doing that.

The main way in which Tosh's visual impairment affected my life was in the respect that I was required to be his informal chauffeur when his reliance on public transport let him down. I never minded. It was nice to have some company. The more pompous elements of our Oxbridge backgrounds came into play as we sang songs while I drove, putting in harmonies as we did so.

One occasion on which my services proved particularly important to Tosh was when he went to dinner with the family of his girlfriend and future wife, Sharon (of whom, more later). I believe that it was the first time that he had met them and dinner was taken at a 'posh' restaurant in Nottingham. Throughout the day, he put regular updates on Facebook and, from a distance, I followed the action. It was Sunday, so I knew that he had to return that night to be ready for work the next morning. Unfortunately, the train would only be able to get him to the city of Peterborough, which was some twenty miles away from his home. Since his vision prevented him from driving, his only option was the X1 bus service.

As the day waned into evening, I changed onto what I described as my 'slobbing around' clothes—leggings, t-shirt, no socks—clothes that could be worn inside, but which were not appropriate to the outdoors. I was getting ready for bed but I continued to monitor Tosh's progress. It was becoming uncomfortably obvious that the meal was not going to take place on schedule. The time at which Tosh had claimed that he would be back in his flat had been passed before he and his party even entered the restaurant.

I changed back into my outdoor clothes, knowing that a call was coming.

Sure enough, at around ten o'clock—the last X1 of the day having long since departed—my mobile rang. I could see on the display that it was Tosh.

'Hi,' I said.

'Mate,' he said, 'Could you give me a lift from Peterborough Station?'

I smirked to myself at my own prescience.

'Sure,' I said, 'Give me about half an hour.'

I set out in my Mazda MX5 (the MR2 was now a thing of the past). The night was cold and the road to Peterborough was more than a little icy. It took me past ploughed fields, petrol stations and strange restaurants—now closed for the night—that had been set up in what was, it must be said, the middle of nowhere. I listened to a bit of music.

It was heavy rock. I needed something to keep me awake.

I found Tosh smoking outside a rather desolate Peterborough Station. There was no one else around. Even the taxi drivers who habitually waited at the edge of the nearby car park had given up and deserted their posts.

Tosh climbed in. As was typical, he acted as though what I was doing was perfectly normal, as though I had gone no further than the next street. He babbled happily about his day, describing the dinner and the company. I was pleased to help, but I did ask him why the party could not have happened in less frosty weather.

As I have already said, Tosh has been my gateway to a whole community of blind and partially sighted people. Some of these were his friends from the specialist school in Worcester that he and they attended. Others were friends of friends and people met through activities aimed at the visually impaired (VI) community. For me, they all helped to put matters into—if the word is apposite—perspective. A couple of Tosh's friends ran an internet radio station. For a long period, I listened to their shows on Sunday afternoons. They were a lot of fun and would always play my requests—I later found out why... Most startling was how little blindness, or near blindness, held those people back. As I increasingly accepted the future as one of growing darkness, Tosh and his friends were living proof that there is no need to be disabled by a disability.

Karen, to speak of her, had the bad luck, or bad timing, to enter my life at around the same time as glaucoma. There is no connection between the two events. I need hardly say that she has been supportive— but that will become clear as this narrative unfolds. Both of these characters—Tosh and Karen—have been, in different ways, the rocks upon which I have built a lighthouse of hope as the disease has made its quiet, often undetected, inroads over the years.

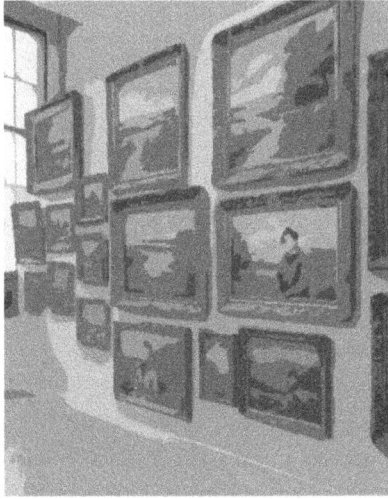

Chapter 4—Just Like Brushing Your Teeth, Really…

NORMALISATION IS THE process of something unusual becoming nothing special. When a new practice is introduced into a person's life soon enough it is just another part of that life. Perhaps the greatest example of normalization that any of us have experienced is the normalisation of the internet. Once exotic and confusing, now so important that we carry it around in our pockets in the form of smartphones. The word 'normalization' is all too often used in a negative sense, as in the normalization of hate/racism/transphobia, but, in its basic form, it is a neutral term that is applied to a process that is, well, normal.

Glaucoma quickly became normalized for me. My fears that I would have to adapt all my routines for it proved to be unfounded. The disease readily accommodated itself to me. I applied the eye drops as part of my morning bathroom business: shit, shave, shower and squirt from the squeezy bottle. In the evening, the eye drops went along with brushing my teeth in readiness for whatever I was planning to do after work. It was another minor inconvenience. If I was going to the cinema, or a party, I could afford to be flexible. It made no real difference if I put in the eye drops early, or a bit late. Sometimes, if I was held up somewhere, I would not put them in until just before I went to bed; that was not ideal, but at least I put them in.

As this process was happening, Sally and I stopped seeing each other (I am aware that, in this book, such phrases serve as both statements of fact and puns). The last experience we shared was going to that hotel in Huntingdon for New Year's Day lunch. It was an unexpectedly grim affair. We had been growing apart for some time. I cannot say why beyond making the bland statement that it happens. The conversation on that occasion was stilted and lacking its customary good humor. We returned to March and that was that. There was never an inquest. We just did not get in touch with each other again.

Almost immediately, I met Karen. That came through scanning the Guardian Soulmates dating ads. I had never really done internet dating but given my age and the limited opportunities for meeting people that it afforded, I had a look online. On a whim, I contacted Karen when I saw that she lived in the reachable city of Nottingham. I was not sure what I expected to gain. Perhaps a single date. Perhaps nothing at all. We arranged to meet in Peterborough—which, lazily, I had told her was about halfway between our homes (it wasn't)—and, to my surprise, hit it off. One encounter turned into another and, before too long, we were in a full-on relationship.

I was honest from the beginning about my eyesight. I needed to be because Karen is as close to embodying physical perfection as it is possible to get. Nothing afflicts her. Bugs and viruses fly around alighting on random members of the population, but they never pick on her. Her blood pressure, resting heart rate and cholesterol are a medical textbook writer's dream. She only started to wear glasses when age caught up with her vision. Telling her about my disease felt like admitting to a tragic flaw.

'I have an eye problem,' I said to her over dinner at an Indian restaurant in Nottingham not long after we met.

'What problem?' she asked.

'Glaucoma.'

'Oh.'

'Do you know what that is?'

'Yes.'

This did not surprise me. She had a broad knowledge of physical afflictions as a result of having cared for her parents for years.

'I have to take eye drops,' I said, 'Twice a day.'

'Okay,' she replied, 'But they might find a cure?'

'I don't know,' I said, 'I'm not sure that even those amazing people called 'they' can beat this one.'

'But you can get on with your life?'

'Of course,' I reassured her, 'It's not that big a deal. I just have to remember to put the drops in.'

That was pretty much the whole discussion. I had been expecting it to be more complicated, but Karen was remarkably unfazed. We carried on spooning curry down our throats and moved on to other interesting and exciting things that we did not know about each other. The relationship had survived a potential early bump.

It continued to grow, even though it was long distance. I was still living in March while she was eighty or so miles up the A1 (a main road) away from me. My week took on a specific shape. I would work at the school. Then, I would either have a drink (followed by a plate of fish and chips) with Tosh on the Friday evening before heading to Nottingham on Saturday morning, or I would head to Nottingham straight after work on Friday, cutting out the food and drink.

Both options overlapped with the Friday evening application of my eye drops. Usually, this did not matter. I would put them in once I arrived home, or upon reaching Nottingham.

Routine, though, can become addiction. It sounds strange, but – like some modern-day Thomas de Quincey - I began to become dependent on taking those drops. I looked forward to the moment when I would put them in, one drop, then, without pause, the other. I started to carry the bottles around, so that I would not have to wait. It must have bemused my fellow customers when, while sitting in a pub or a café or a restaurant, I would whisk out a bottle, throw back my head and shoot the soothing cool drops of Travatan, then Azarga, at my parched eyeballs.

That I was getting ever closer to Karen was demonstrated by my inviting her to my PhD graduation at Birmingham University a few months after we started to see each other. I was allowed two guest tickets. She got one, my Mum the other. As events go, it was certainly visually spectacular. In that respect, it was a reminder of how much eysight is to be treasured. I am not sure whether it was the last time that I wore contact lenses; it was close to the last, for sure. To some extent, the decision to ditch the lenses was just born of indolence. Wearing them can be more trouble than it's worth. Putting the things in and getting them out is a nuisance, but they are also another source of anxiety. As soon as they go in, the countdown to their eventual removal begins. As the hours pass, they become less and less comfortable. Pulling them out and placing them in the nearest bin is another source of relief. Having an excuse to do away with them forever was among the few benefits of glaucoma.

The appointments with the eye doctor continued. Fields tests. Scans. Pressure checks. For a while, my eyes behaved themselves. The pressures remained at a 'safe' level. So much so, indeed, that, once, I went for a whole year without visiting the clinic and, when I did, I was looked after by a nurse practitioner, not the doctor. This I took as a good sign. The degree of risk to my sight must have been downgraded, I conjectured. I was in a treatment holding pattern. The drops were working and everything seemed to be going fine.

Nevertheless, I longed for some more permanent solution. Returning to a life that did not include eye drops was the Holy Grail. I had been told by various opticians and ophthalmologists that a lot of research was being done into glaucoma and that breakthroughs were always possible. The March doctor mentioned one possibility: an operation.

'Can you do that?' I asked, knowing that he was a surgeon primarily. Indeed, we had already discussed the oddness of my being called 'Dr' despite not working as a doctor, whereas he was not 'Dr' even though he did work as one: surgeons are always called 'Mr' for historical reasons related to professional pride.

'Oh yes,' he said, 'Glaucoma operations are the most common type that I do.'

'What does it involve?'

'Well, basically, I would put a trap door in the top of your eyeball that allows the excess fluid out.'

This sounded a little gruesome.

'Where does the fluid go?' I probed, uncertainty in my voice.

'Oh, just into your body. It is totally harmless.'

I thought about this.

One operation and everything would be okay?

That sounded like a pretty sweet deal.

'Why don't I just do that?' I suggested.

He shook his head.

'Operations are a bit of a last resort. Most people I do them on are quite old. Invasive interventions always carry some risk, however slight. We prefer to use drops if we can.'

'Fair enough,' I said.

Even so, a seed had been planted.

My interest was not purely about wishing to beat the disease. I knew that it was unbeatable. The best that I could hope for was some kind of neutralization of it. But I used my eyes a lot. I know that we all do, but the visual dimension was crucial not only to my job, but to many of my interests in life. As an English teacher, being able to read was very important, for a start.

I was always fond of answering the question, 'how do you incorporate information technology into your lessons', with the answer, 'in my subject, information technology means a book.' It was a jokey line, but, for people with limited vision, it conceals a harsher truth. The lighting in classrooms is never especially helpful. Neon-generated and bleaching, it causes the dull grey of a page to be difficult to read at the best of times. Add to that small font sizes and making out anything from the page of a study text can be difficult even for those with excellent vision. I was still able to read everything without a problem, but I was acutely conscious of the fact that, as my sight became increasingly poor, I would need to hold books ever closer to my face until they hid it completely. What that would mean for my relationship with my pupils and—more seriously—my ability to keep order in the room was yet to be revealed. Again, I took inspiration from Tosh: he was in exactly that position but coped.

Not that he did not have hurdles to overcome. Recognising students and putting a face to a name had always been difficult for him. On one occasion with his previous employer, this had caused him, at a parents' evening, to send a straight-A Oxbridge candidate away in floods of tears after he had mistaken her for a less high-achieving member of her class and not held back on the—constructive—criticism. Another time, he led with 'Suzanne is doing really well in French,' only to learn that he was speaking to the parents of Emma, who did not do the subject. On a day-to-day basis, he did not look forward to group work, which can be a nightmare to organise for fully-sighted teachers with co-operative students. Name tags on lanyards were useless to him: in order to read them, he would have had to get so close to a person that he would have been in court quicker than you could say, 'Jimmy Saville'.

He told me that his strategy was to compensate for his disability with force of personality. Humour worked, as in the Suzanne/Emma debacle, but he was aware that, in some classroom environments, pupils were likely to take advantage of his condition—as, much later, they did during a day's supply work at an academy in Nottingham that can only be described as 'torrid'. Being up front with pupils had always served him well, slightly patronising shows of support being the usual response.

His biggest challenge has never been doing the job so much as landing it in the first place, many headteachers being somewhat nervous about employing someone with his disability. A case in point was an interview for a position for which he was the only candidate, a situation that, in his words, was 'unfuckupable'. It was an open goal! Asking for feedback having not been appointed, he was given the totally contrived answer that his sample lesson had been 'pitched too high'. As Tosh has said, disabled people generally have to do much more than their fully abled counterparts if they want to get a job offer.

Tosh, Karen and I were not frequently together as a group, but one occasion that does stand out was when we all went to see the rock band

Status Quo perform in the city of Birmingham. This is worth mentioning because 'see' is probably not the most apposite verb. We went to hear them play. Karen and I picked Tosh up in Karen's car—which was more like a van with back seats—and headed to the West Midlands from Cambridgeshire. It was a chilly day, but we were anticipating an excellent night, especially as the support act were none other than Chas & Dave, a duo who performed a brand of piano-led good time bar room style music that they had self-titled 'Rockney' in honour of its—and their—London roots. It was a gig by two bands who were both almost ridiculously entertaining. What was not to like?

One thing was the potential volume. I did not expect Chas & Dave to be too ear-splitting, but Status Quo had a reputation for being insanely loud. I had been to many a rock concert before and was aware that my hearing was certainly not what it had once been. If my eyesight was disappearing, did I really want to risk further damage to a sense that I might need to rely on in the future? I expressed my worries to Tosh as we passed through Peterborough.

'I wouldn't worry about it, mate,' he said, 'You'll probably get to the Big Sleep before it becomes too serious.'

'Yes,' I said, drily, 'I hadn't thought of that...'

We arrived in Birmingham early in the day and left the car at an extremely expensive car park close to the Arena in which the concert was to be held. We had resolved to take advantage of the Christmas Market that had been installed in the centre of the city, although 'market' barely does it justice. 'Small-wooden-town-within-the-city' might be a better term. Stretching from the bottom of New Street—the main shopping area—through the Central Library (as it then was) and on to Centenary Square—which was close to the Arena—it rivaled anything similar in Germany, where such things had been invented. Its edge was marked by a temporary Ferris Wheel, which gave spectacular views of the city while offering a recorded commentary in French that referred to landmarks in Paris. A subplot to this odd state of affairs was that when the recording was changed to one in English that was actually about Birmingham, it proved so unpopular with customers that the Paris one was quickly reinstated.

Vile Jelly

At the market, we had a cup of that not conspicuously English drink Gluhwein to stave off the chill. Tosh and I also had a couple of bratwursts that were long enough to make even the most blessed of stallions blush. Eventually, the time came to repair to the arena for the gig.

As with all such venues, the cavernous performance space was surrounded by corridors in which were located the toilets, bars, food outlets and, crucially, merch sellers. We had a beer and then took our seats at the back of the arena. We were not to be seated for long.

Chas & Dave came on. Despite their name, they were basically a trio: pianist, bass guitarist and drummer.

'You're going to have a great night!' Chas announced.

They launched into their first song. It was immediately apparent that they were not going to disappoint. By the time they reached their finale, the evergreen classic, *Ain't No Pleasing You*, Tosh and I were converts (Karen was less sure).

'I'm going to get one of their t-shirts!' Tosh said, enthusiastically.

'Fuck yeah!' I said, reinforcing his zeal.

'I am definitely a fan!' Tosh went on.

We went back out to the main thoroughfare during the break between acts and bought t-shirts that were white with the band's logo wedged between two drawn-on braces (this being emblematic of their 'Cockney' image). We changed in a toilet and were ready for the main act, albeit that we were not exactly attired for it.

I was generally feeling quite optimistic regarding my hearing. Chas & Dave's volume had been more than acceptable. My ears were not buzzing. I could envisage a future in which gigs would not be a problem, irrespective of what might be happening to my eyes.

Back in the auditorium, a large cyclorama had been draped across the stage. The lights dimmed. For a moment, the space was in darkness. Then a solitary spotlight, behind the sheet, picked out the silhouette of a man, legs akimbo, guitar in hand, thrashing out the opening riff to Status Quo's hit, *Caroline*. Tosh later confessed that he was not able to see this at all. This was not unusual. He was never able to see what was happening on stage at any gig. He was only able to identify any given band or band member by the music and his general knowledge of who was playing. And for Quo, he could certainly hear them. As could I, Karen and the packed audience that rose as one to their feet with a cheer as the riff started.

If my hope had been that the volume would not be significantly higher than it had been for Chas and Dave, I was given a rapid reality check. It was loud. Deafeningly loud. When the rest of the band joined in, it was as though a shock wave of noise spread out over the audience, blasting out ear drums and nearly knocking me off my feet.

'Shit,' I said to no one who could pick up my words, 'I wish that I had bought some of those noise reducing ear plugs now!'

But with a rock concert on this scale, there was nothing to do but go with it. I knew, for example, that the first two or three songs would be fairly crisp and clear, but, thereafter, everything would flatten out into a tsunami of undifferentiated sound, deadening whatever subtleties the music contained (to be fair, these were in relatively short supply with Status Quo's repertoire). By the inevitable encores, any connection between my inner ear and the world from which it was supposed to be gathering information would be through the medium of a muffling blanket.

As we left the arena at the end of what had been—all caveats aside—a thoroughly enjoyable gig, I asked Tosh what he thought.

'Fucking brilliant mate!' Was his reply.

Karen gave a more guarded, 'It was good.'

After a couple of days, my—and I guess Tosh and Karen's—hearing was back to normal. Probably. I suppose you never really know. I could have lost my capacity to discern a whole range of sounds. I would get used to it.

In terms of my senses taking a battering, my other main concern was around art. I have always averred that the thing I am best at is drawing and painting. I'm quite a good writer, I would say, but art is my God-given talent. In the pre-glaucoma days, I had stumbled over a crate onto a concrete floor and completely smashed up my drawing arm. There is still a foot-long metal plate in there. Needless to say, I lost much of my supination: that did not bother me as such, but I was terrified that it might affect my drawing. Fortunately, it did not, but glaucoma presented an even greater threat. If I cannot see, I cannot draw.

My response was to tough it out and I became remarkably productive for a while. Political cartoons, four panel comic strips, pastel drawings based on ancient legends, portraits—for a while, I churned out new pieces as though it were a full-time job. I used pens, paper, crayons, my iPad. When I put on a school production of the Queen jukebox musical *We Will Rock You*, I produced a number of backdrops with pens and acrylic paints that were projected onto a cyclorama at the back of the stage.

I continued to enjoy art as an observer. A frequent excursion would be to London to meet my friend Loz for what we called a 'gallery day'. This meant visiting several art galleries and assorted exhibitions in between coffees, lunch and afternoon tea. Did I notice my appreciation of the paintings and sculptures that we viewed reducing as my eyesight went? Not really. Beyond short-sightedness, nothing seemed amiss. The colours were as bright as ever—so I thought—the lines as sharp. It was business as usual.

But, as I stared at some piece of pretentious silliness that Loz had tried to convince me was 'brilliant', glaucoma was never off my mind. I was always making a mental calculation: does this look the same as it would have this time last week, or yesterday, or this morning? What if I close one eye? Better? Or worse? Do the lines look as straight? That slight fuzziness—was it there last time I looked at a painting on a wall? Is there even a fuzziness there? Am I mistaken?

It was at such moments that it occurred to me that I was in a perpetual state of self-diagnosis. Every time I opened my eyes, I was taking a sample of my vision and subjecting it to analysis. I was not doing so as an expert, that was true, but no one had greater insight into what I could physically see than I did. Was there a noticeable change? Was the world darkening and closing in around me? I could never be entirely certain. All I could do was carry on accepting it for what it was and hoping.

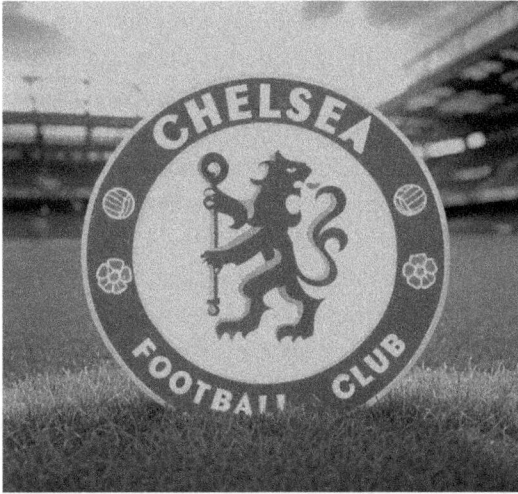

Chapter 5—The One-Eyed Man

THE EYE IS a marvel of evolution. It might even be proof that there is no such thing as evolution and that everything in the world was created, after all, in a flash of inspiration by a benign—if oddly shy—superbeing. That is not just me talking: Charles Darwin himself considered the eye to be the inconvenient fact that made him doubt the validity of his signature theory. He was right. Think about it. How does something so unlikely appear ex nihilo, or even develop over time from the workings of impersonal and random forces? Think about what the eye can do. Think about what we mean by 'seeing'.

The question is not so much how did we end up with the eye, but what were the interim stages on the way from it not existing to its being the precision piece of natural engineering that it is today? Presumably, the most primitive creatures were blind. How much vision do you really need if you are not much more than a sponge-like piece of matter floating around at the bottom of the ocean? What, then, was stage one of the eye's development? Photosensitive cells? Perhaps, but where did they come from? And what did they do next? Did they become a bit more photosensitive? At what point did they cease to be just a few cells and turn into something as mind-bogglingly complex as an eye?

According to Trevor Lamb in Scientific American [1] , the intermediate stages may not be quite as mysterious as everyone, including Darwin, may have thought. Apparently, something called a hagfish still possesses what might be the most primitive version of the eye. As an organ for seeing, it is not very effective, but since a hagfish is one of those proto-lifeforms that exists exclusively to ingest stuff, spectacular vision is not one of its big needs. Anyway, it proves, or strongly suggests, that the eye evolved at least five hundred million years ago at a point at which living organisms split off into those with insect-style 'compound eyes' and those, like, eventually, us, that are blessed with the more sophisticated 'camera eyes'. This certainly explains why the eye is so ubiquitous. Apart from creatures—moles for example—whose evolution rather unluckily involved the loss of them, pretty much everything in nature has eyes. Most are not unlike ours. A cat has an eye that differs very little from that of a human, except in being far better at its job.

The upshot of all this is that we should make sure that we look after our eyes. They may be the universe's masterpiece. But it is by no means always the case that we do look after them. We use them to squint at radiation-emitting computer screens, we drip shampoo into them, poke them, rub them and generally take them far more for granted than we should. I suppose a positive effect of glaucoma was to make me starkly aware of what I had and what I stood to lose.

This will come as cold comfort to those who have lost their fight already—or who never had the chance to wage it in the first place. In the land of the blind, the saying goes, the one-eyed man is king. At some stages of his life, that made Tosh king. At his school for the visually impaired in Worcester, he was mostly around children who were totally blind and he had better vision than the majority of those who were partially sighted. At a school in Bradford, also supposedly for the visually

---

[1] Lamb, T. (2011). *Evolution of the Eye*. Scientific American, https://www.scientificamerican.com/article/evolution-of-the-eye/ [accessed Sunday 12th November 2023].

impaired, he had some of the worst vision and so became known as the 'blind kid'. That in later life he was given lifts in cars by some of his erstwhile classmates from there says a lot.

For some reason, Tosh and I called our Friday evening after-work pub—which was located in Wisbech—'The Witch's Legs', although that was not its real name. We had something of an unresolved—and unresolvable—debate about whether this imaginary soubriquet was *Witch's* singular, or *Witches'* plural. The older guy behind the bar, who was not the owner, quickly acquired the nickname 'Speedy Gonzalez'. This was on account of his general lack of urgency and energy. Despite Tosh and I invariably being his only customers, our orders would take an age to be served. They generally came with a whole lot of moaning about how hard the job of serving them was. Weirdly, the beer barrels almost always needed to be changed, even though there was no plausible explanation for why the current ones should have run out in the first place. Barrel-changing called for Speedy to vacate the bar for long periods during which Tosh and I would hang around in an increasingly Pinteresque state of existential doubt.

My conversations with Tosh at the Witch's—or Witches'—would often turn to eyes. I found out more about the limits of Tosh's vision, which only increased my admiration for his levels of independence. I learned about the VI community, which began almost to seem like a slightly exotic subculture, with its own communication networks and jargon. I learned, for example, that those who were completely blind were known as 'totals' and people like Tosh 'partials'. It was while discussing such things that Tosh announced that he might be about to find himself in a relationship. The woman in question lived down south somewhere—close to London, I believe. She and Tosh had got talking online via mutual VI friends. He told me about her one evening in the Witch's.

'What's her name?' I asked.

'Sharon,' he replied, adding, 'I think she's into me, mate.'

'Really?' I said.

'Yes! We were talking for over two hours on the phone last night.'

'Wow! I am not sure that I have ever been on the phone for two hours with a woman!'

'The only problem is that she's a Chelsea fan,' Tosh said.

For many, this would be a light-hearted throwaway comment. Not so Tosh. As a lifelong, ardent, fan of Liverpool football club, these things mattered to him. He was particularly scathing of clubs, such as Chelsea, that could plausibly have been accused of buying their success.

'Well, I'm sure that you can get over that,' I said.

I decided to take a pot shot at the elephant in the room.

'Is she—you know—' I began.

'She's blind,' he confirmed, 'she's a total.'

'That's not a problem, is it?' I ventured.

'Not at all!' he said.

A meeting at her place was arranged for as soon as was convenient for both of them. An excited Tosh marked the date in his calendar and booked a train ticket. But then disaster struck. While plugging in his phone charger—an operation that required him to crouch—he fell over and injured his foot.

At school the next day, he showed me what he was trying to sell as a bruise. I have broken a toe before now and so know what to look out for. He had definitely broken a toe.

'You'd better get to the quack, mate,' I counseled.

'No, no, it'll be fine. It's just a bruise.'

I knew why he was saying that—he did not want to cancel his trip—but there's not much hiding from reality when your foot is so swollen that it no longer fits inside your shoe.

'That is definitely not just a bruise,' I said, 'Do you need a lift to the surgery?'

He declined that offer but was sensible enough to get himself to the hospital in the afternoon. When I next saw him, he was wearing the kind of heavy plastic foot brace that looks like an imperial stormtrooper's boot and commonly goes under the informal name of 'pot'. I was surprised to walk into the staff room and see him there.

'What the fuck are you doing here?' I asked.

'Working,' was his simple response.

'I can see that,' I said, 'but aren't you supposed to be at home resting?'

'The doctor said I should,' he explained, 'but I said, you're joking aren't you? I've got a full timetable and mock orals to do. I can't sit around at home scratching my arse.'

I said nothing, but he was not fooling me—and he knew that he was not fooling me and I knew that he knew that he was not fooling me. He knew that he could hardly honour his commitment to head south if he was off work. So he had disregarded medical advice and turned up to hobble around like a badly carved toy soldier in order to pre-empt any awkward questions about why he was not well enough to come to work but had no problem with catching a string of buses and trains to see his putative girlfriend. Again, his grit was not in doubt.

While Tosh was working on his love life, I was moving to Wisbech. My newly acquired home was a flat on the top floor of a redeveloped Victorian warehouse, a loft apartment—or loft penthouse, as more than one estate agent spun it. Karen helped me move, a task that, among other things, involved the two of us lugging a very heavy coffee table made from reclaimed wood up five flights of stairs.

The place was lovely, with antique wooden beams criss-crossing the large, open plan main room and slick, glossy built-in wardrobes in the master bedroom. The bare brick walls were luxurious in context. The crowning glory was a small balcony overlooking both the block's gardens and the Nene, which was the river that flowed through the town in a not especially picturesque way.

Wisbech was a good example of an English town. Some parts of it—including the one that I lived in—were achingly beautiful. A part of the centre known as the Crescent was smaller than its namesake in Bath, but no less delightful, being a ring of perfectly preserved Georgian townhouses. The 'Brinks' that lined the river were an anthology of architectural gems, ranging from Medieval Rustic to Palladian. For all that, it was not a wealthy town and much of it had a rundown and sorry look about it. It was also not entirely urban, but not entirely rural either. There were a few factories here and there, mostly concerned with the processing of food, but the countryside and farming were never far away. Right next to the school, which was more-or-less central, were corn fields. My new walk to work—along a street just behind the main shopping area—took me past a paddock full of sheep. Wherever you stood, you were never more than a few minutes' amble away from agricultural land.

It was on a field at the edge of town that someone decided to build ACES, the headquarters for Anglia Community Eye Service, an establishment that was to become almost my second home over the next few years. Named for the fact that it was in Cambridgeshire, which is in East Anglia, it seemed to have been envisaged as part of a major development that was to encompass a large new supermarket, a cinema and other leisure facilities. A sign about this went up not long after I arrived in the area (in the pre-glaucoma days), only for the 2008 financial crisis to almost immediately hit. For years, that sign remained in situ, becoming ever more drab, weathered and irrelevant. When, at last, the development did occur, it looked not much like the sketch on the sign.

Happily, ACES, being publicly funded, went ahead irrespective of the ravages of sub-prime mortgages. An intriguing structure began to take shape. The main block was dominated by a huge arched window. I wondered what might lie behind it. My imagination conjured up chapels, open-plan offices, even some kind of college. It was a while before I found out.

It was not built quickly—it grew at roughly the pace of Petrocelli's house. Bits would appear and then everything would go quiet. Then a roof went on. And everything went quiet. The car park was laid. Then everything went quiet…you get the picture. Once the structure was completed, everything went quiet. Presumably, the interior was being fitted. Whatever—a lengthy interval passed without any sign that an opening was imminent.

In the meantime, I was settling in and getting used to my new life in the town. The best thing about it was that I was walking distance from just about everything. The Witch's Legs was so close that I could see it from my balcony. Two excellent chip shops (one run by a guy called Adrian Jarvis, the other that which Tosh and I frequented) could be reached and returned from before any procured take away food had lost its heat. The Market Square was just across the river. Wisbech was far from a large town, but living in the centre of it conferred considerable benefits.

Close to my block's entrance was a coffee house called Café D'Light. I always found this a little bemusing, since the spelling did not only fail to save any syllables when the name was spoken but was not even more thrifty to write. Why not just go with 'delight' and be done with it? Ah well, it was, to be fair, a nice hang out that served good, inexpensive, food and pleasant hot drinks. It also always had a couple of tables set up on the pavement outside. These afforded one of the best views in town, of the Dickens-adaptation film location that was Old Market and the Town Bridge that spanned the Nene and brought the two Brinks together. Tosh and I got into the habit of sitting at those tables for half an hour or so after work to have a drink and chat.

Among our favourite topics was Tosh's burgeoning romance. Sharon—his by-now girlfriend—had been married before and had three adult daughters, all of whom were sighted. Tosh referred to her ex as her 'first husband'. I misunderstood this at first.

'Has she been married more than once, then?' I asked, sipping my latte.

'No,' he hastily covered, 'I mean her ex-husband.'

I looked at him a little askance. He and Sharon had not been together all that long. There was a clear implication to his words.

'Tosh,' I began, 'Have you talked about getting married to her?"

He puffed on his roll up.

'We've talked about options,' he said.

I imagined that marriage was one of those options. It was another little insight into the VI world. I am sure that there are many, many VI people who are happily married to people who enjoy perfect vision but membership of the VI community must narrow the pool of eligible partners. This is not in any way to endorse ableism, but, realistically, it must make a difference. Tosh had had fully sighted girlfriends before, but he always seemed to be at his most comfortable around others with visual impairments. As for Sharon, she faced the double whammy of visual impairment and having a grown-up family. Both were restrictions on what she could accept or commit herself to. A few long phone calls and a couple of meetings must have seemed like enough for a preliminary decision to be taken. After all, one motive for getting together would be to guarantee mutual help and support. I knew that Tosh was a caring and considerate guy. Sharon was lucky to have found him in that respect.

She came not only with a family but a guide dog. Tosh professed a great love of dogs. He was going to need it because that dog was shortly to get him into all kinds of trouble.

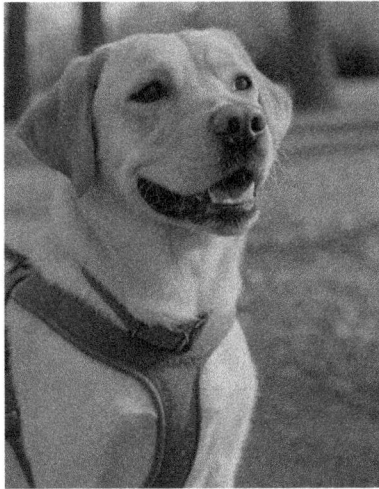

Chapter 6—Lasers and Labradors

ON SEVERAL OCCASIONS, I found myself in Nottingham on a Saturday with no eye drops. This would happen for one of two reasons. Either I would simply forget to take them with me when I went up to visit Karen, or I would squeeze a bottle into my eyes, only to discover it was empty. Appreciating that these might seem like the actions of someone suffering from monumental levels of stupidity, I can only say that they are much easier to do than might be imagined.

As I have said, the main problem that I have faced over the years with regard to putting in eye drops is remembering whether or not I have done it at all. When something becomes so much a part of your life, it only registers with the short-term memory. It disappears from the consciousness almost immediately. Even ten minutes later, it becomes next-to-impossible to remember whether or not it has happened. There was little point in trying to come up with some mnemonic to make certain: I would invariably forget that, too. Someone who can forget his own mnemonic cannot be blamed too harshly for sometimes forgetting to take his eye drops with him on a journey.

Unexpectedly running out of the things may seem like an even more dunderheaded thing to do. Can't you just check by looking? The answer is no. The bottles are opaque and shaking them provides no reliable information. They sound full of liquid right up to the point at which they contain no liquid at all. Ensuring a steady supply, then, became a constant hassle.

It was made more difficult than it needed to be by the fact that the drops were prescription drugs. They could not be obtained without a doctor's sign off. And, usually, not just any doctor: the patient's own GP had to be the one (as I was to find, this was not a hard-and-fast rule, but breaking it meant turning into a character from a Kafka novel).

Fortunately, it was possible to register with an online system that allowed repeat prescriptions—my eye drops certainly fell into that category—to be requested without the need to go into the doctor's surgery. Foresight was, however, required. If the medicine was requested too early, it would simply be refused. So, it needed to be requested long enough before the previous lot ran out to maintain continuity of supply, but not too long as to cause the doctor to send the request back with words equivalent to 'nice try but come back later'.

After moving to Wisbech, I remained, for a while, registered with the doctor in March, which meant returning there whenever I needed to pick up a prescription. The pharmacy was attached to the doctor's surgery and had an oddly comforting air about it. Yes, I know that pharmacists work hard, but I have always found their places of work welcoming and rather cosy. Perhaps it is because walking into one is to be instantly surrounded by things that cure, heal and sustain life. Perhaps it is the general air of calm and purposefulness. Perhaps it is that so many are open until late and shine out on otherwise dark streets, sometimes proclaiming themselves with those continental-style green illuminated crosses, like havens of love and care in a harsh world.

I would generally go to the Pharmacy in March after work, leave my car in the surgery car park and go in wearing my work clothes, making the pharmacist's invariable query about whether I paid for prescriptions somewhat redundant: I was clearly earning too much to get them for free. I must confess that I had ready a whole repertoire of sarcastic answers for when the question was put to me: 'Well, I'm dressed like this, so what do you think?' was one; 'Yep! I'm the one!' was another; 'Yes, but one day, I'll be retired and then it will be someone else's turn,' was yet another. None of these, I would stress, were because I resented having to pay. I did, obviously, but not that much. I always resisted cutting my bill by buying an up-front certificate on the grounds that I could afford it and the NHS was worth supporting.

Still, those times that I turned up in Nottingham not properly supplied proved that the system could work to my advantage. What to do? It was always too late to call my GP. Fortunately, there was an emergency line that would issue a prescription for whichever of the drops I was lacking. There were two possible suppliers that I could go to. One was called Latenight Pharmacy. It did not quite live up to its name because I think that it closed around 9pm, but it was the archetype of the 'beacon of hope' variety. It was on a main road in an area that was not conspicuously salubrious and which was very quiet after dark. Inside, there was a counter that was open on all sides next to which were a few steps leading up to the area, a couple of metres above, in which prescriptions were prepared—this always reminded me of some kind of altar.

The other option was probably the most impressive dispenser of medicines that I have ever encountered. Located in the Hyson Green area of Nottingham, it was less a shop than a depot. Along the entire length of one side was a counter that a tank would have had trouble driving through. Behind this was shelf after shelf, drawer after drawer, cabinet after cabinet, of pills, potions and ointments.

It must have stocked every medicine ever devised.

Unlike Latenight Pharmacy, it was not staffed by a couple of young women, but a whole army of people in white coats. It was open late. I'm not sure that it ever closed. If a prescription request was sent there from the emergency line, I was confident that I would be able to get whatever it was that I needed. The downside was that it was the exception to the rule about pharmacies being nice places to be. It was not horrible, but it was a little too industrial, a little too neon-lit. Yes, it was efficient, but, sometimes, the more friendly environment of Latenight Pharmacy was more to my liking.

Either way, I could source my drops. A felicitous side effect was that I would often end up with something of a surfeit as the emergency supply supplemented the drops that waited for me back in Wisbech. All of this, it must be said, happened before the COVID pandemic came along and turned the world upside down.

By now, Tosh was well into his relationship. Friday nights at the Witch's were mostly a thing of the past. He would rush out of school at the end of the working week to get the X1 bus to Peterborough Station from where he would catch the earliest London train possible. His mind tended to work that way: bullet-like focus on a single activity, rather than juggling several at once.

Since guide dogs were now a main feature of his life, he became a big advocate for them and their owners. For those who may not know, a guide dog is an animal trained to lead blind and visually impaired people around the town or city in which they happen to live. This does not make of them some kind of organic satnav, but they know to stop at curbs and when to cross a road safely. They have the ancillary function of providing their owners with both companionship and protection, since they are always labradors or German shepherds. I have never seen a member of that breed that look like hippy rats working as a guide dog. Guide dogs are trained and provided by a charity, although, once donated, they fall under the ownership of the human being to whom they are providing assistance.

Tosh and Sharon gave a talk at the school one evening on the subject of guide dogs. The audience learned about how the dogs were selected, trained and what happened to them once they had reached the end of their period of service: they could either be returned to the Guide Dog Association for rehousing, or kept as pets. Tosh suggested that he and Sharon would go down the latter route with her current dog. Sharon was less sentimental. I more than once witnessed her being quite critical of its abilities. That is not to say that there was not a bond, but owner and dog have to be partners: that dog lacked confidence and was often rather timid in performing its duties. In the end, it was returned prior to the end of its usefulness and replaced, although this was less to do with its abilities than Sharon's concerns around how well she would bond with her new dog if the old one were still hanging around. The parting was not without some tears—from Tosh, too.

As part of that school session, Sharon demonstrated her dexterity with Braille, the alphabet that uses a collection of raised dots in patterns that can be 'read' with the fingertips as a substitute for letters that require vision. She had a machine—a sort of Braille Kindle—that sent through 'words' in a loop. Her reading speed was incredibly high—at least matching that of a sighted person.

Afterwards, another colleague said to me of Sharon, 'Remarkable lady,' with a supercilious smirk.

Patronising as she was, she was at least well-meaning, which was not something that could be said of everyone. Discrimination against guide dogs and, by extension, their owners, was rife. Some of it came from those in the general population who—like me—were anything but dog lovers. Unfortunately, it was also very much a feature of tradesmen and women with whom members of the VI community might come into contact.

Taxi could be particularly difficult environments. Tosh's VI circle frequently clogged up my Facebook timeline with links to a story about some driver or other refusing to take a guide dog into their car. A couple of Tosh's VI friends were known to take such people to court, winning appropriate damages, while doing nothing to change the practices that had engendered their actions. At stake was the application of the Equality Act.

It is important to understand this piece of legislation. Passed in 2010, it created so-called 'protected groups', such as women, ethnic minorities, people with particular sexual orientations, transgender people and disabled people. The aim was to enshrine in law the principle of equity. This differs from equality in being to do with 'levelling the playing field' between individuals. Rather than simply saying that everyone has the same rights and opportunities, it acknowledges that some people need extra help simply to get to the starting point for equality. It would be wrong to say that the Act has been free of controversy.

On the whole, however, VI people were not the ones causing it.

Life was tough enough without picking fights—unless you were Tosh. Pugnacious by nature, he took to carrying around a card that reinforced his and Sharon's rights under the 2010 Act and which could be presented when they were challenged (it was not always read by those to whom it was shown).

It came into play during an unfortunate incident in an Indian restaurant that Tosh and I had used many times, although I will say no more about its location than that. As anyone living in the UK will know, 'Indian' restaurants are not really Indian as such. Almost all of them are actually Bangladeshi in origin and, indeed, cuisine. This is a fine distinction, since Bangladesh was carved out of a chunk of what was once India, but it does mean that dogs are not usually popular with those running the restaurants. Something else that was not far from being Bangladeshi in origin was Tosh, as evidenced by his Bengali name.

He had tried to enter the restaurant before with a guide dog and been turned away, which had occasioned much indignation and swearing on his part. On the night of the incident, he went in armed not only with his documentation but a couple of friends—the better to reinforce the rights of Sharon and her guide dog.

I was not there. The first I heard about what happened was when I saw something on Facebook. Tosh did not hold back. He had been told that he was not allowed in and an argument had broken out. It became heated. The Facebook post was accompanied with a Trip Advisor review which gave by far the most complete account of what had transpired:

> *I have thoroughly enjoyed dining at this restaurant in the past (at no small expense) but could scarcely believe how they treated my blind girlfriend and me this evening, denying us entry because of her guide dog. They were deaf to our attempts to point out that they were in default of the 2010 Equality Act; the owner refused outright to read the official ADUK documentation that we carried, instead declaring that he, 'did not have to give a reason' for his attitude. That cliché is intended to allow proprietors to bar entry to people likely to behave*

*inappropriately, not to discriminate against those who
are disabled or members of any other protected group.
Moreover, that they withdrew our reservation—made
twenty four hours earlier—when they discovered that a
guide dog would be present did indeed constitute a
reason, although the manager was coy about saying so.
We called the police, who did not enforce the criminal
law, although they did advise us to pursue a civil claim.
This is precisely our proposed course of action, along with
involving our local MP and the press.*

I spoke to Tosh the next day.

'What on earth happened?' I asked, incredulous.

He explained, finishing: 'They're fucked! They've broken the law!'

I felt inclined to play devil's advocate.

'It's a private business. They can serve whoever they like.'

But Tosh made the good point that:

'Private business, yes! But public space. The 2010 act applies.'

I was not sure what to say. I was sympathetic to Tosh and Sharon but wondered what they could realistically do.

Tosh gave his take.

'We're sending a legal letter. Bastards! It's blatant discrimination!'

'True,' I said, largely to be supportive.

The situation quickly escalated. A letter to the local newspaper went unpublished and unanswered, but the local MP replied to the one he received, although only to say that, as an individual in the House of Commons, his influence was limited.

As for the civil case, I did not read any of Tosh's paperwork, but I was shown the rather astounding communication that he got back from the restaurant's lawyers.

'They're claiming that I was the one being banned, not the dog!' he told me one evening at the Witch's.

I was amazed at this.

'Really?'

'Yes,' he said, 'they're saying that I had been in on other occasions drunk and rowdy and that they didn't want me in there.'

One half of this was, to be fair, sort-of true. I had been into the restaurant with Tosh after a few beers and he had been a little inebriated, but he had never been disruptive. He had once fallen, rather dramatically, off a chair in the middle of a mouthful of Vindaloo, but that had happened at a different restaurant and he had been sober at the time. Generally, the worst that he could be accused of was swearing, but not such as to be a public nuisance.

I perused the letter. Not only did it cast a number of aspersions on Tosh's character, but it suggested that he had gone to the restaurant on the fateful night spoiling for a fight. It questioned his carrying documentation around the 2010 Act, arguing that it was clear evidence of his malign intent; why else, would someone carry around such material? If they had asked me, I would have confirmed that it was entirely in character. It must be said that the letter was worded as strongly as Tosh's trip advisor review.

'Oh,' I said, somewhat non-plussed, 'what are you going to do now?'

'Not much I can do, mate,' he said, 'It's my word against theirs. There's nothing to stop them banning me.'

The whole affair demonstrated how tough life can be for people with visual impairments. Not being one of the more vocal minority groups, they are prone to being ignored. The restaurant cannot be entirely blamed. In spite of what some people may believe, it is not obligatory in the UK to love dogs and they were a place that served food—which does not go well with live animals. But guide dogs are something of an exception. It should be noted that relevant cultural organizations have declared that rules about dogs being unclean are to be waived in the case of guide dogs—making the whole dispute somewhat unnecessary.

For me, the big news was the long-anticipated opening of ACES. My treatment was immediately transferred there and I never again met the smartly dressed doctor in March. Now I was in the hands of several practitioners. The one I saw most often was an Eastern European woman who did her job with a seriousness verging on the dour. Whereas the smartly dressed guy had always stressed the positives, she was inclined to be less upbeat.

During one not especially noteworthy check-up (nothing much to report: pressures fine, fields not altered), she announced quite casually that my eyesight would deteriorate so rapidly and completely that I would have to give up driving soon. This was not what I wanted to hear since I had only recently bought the MX5.

On the whole, though, things were going quite well. My pressures were always at an acceptable level and so my prescription did not change. ACES was not exactly just around the corner from my flat, but it was no more than a twenty-minute walk away. I was obliged to go there on foot because my appointment letters stressed that I might have something done that would blur my vision for long enough to make driving home dangerous. This never really happened, but I did not mind, since it gave me the chance to take a little exercise. I would sometimes cross the road after an appointment to have a coffee in the branch of a chain café that occupied part of the new supermarket. I recall phoning Karen on one occasion to deliver the good news that everything was fine, that I could get on with my life, that I would see her next weekend...

Then, during a visit to ACES, I discovered that everything was not fine.

The arched window proved to be part of a large room—a hall really—that housed the reception and a waiting area. I was sitting there when I happened to notice on a door in the corridor that went off from it a sign that had not been there before. It said words to the effect that caution was to be exercised when entering the room behind because it housed—I was not sure that I read this correctly—a laser.

There is nothing novel about laser eye surgery. It has been a thing for a long time. Aimed at returning twenty-twenty vision to those with myopia, it involves shaving layers off the cornea. It is conventionally provided by the private sector. I was not aware that the NHS offered the procedure. Beyond mild interest, I paid scant attention to the sign and got back to reading the news on my phone.

I was called through and went into the doctor's room. It contained her desk, a chair for the patient and various pieces of machinery for probing the eyes.

'Let's have a look,' she said with no preamble.

She put some yellow dye into my eyes and moved a light in front of me, ordering me to look at her ears in turn as she did so. I rested my chin on the usual machine's pad to get the pressures checked. She 'mmm-ed' as she did so.

'Nice weather,' I said.

'Mmm,' she said.

The examination complete, I sat back.

'Nineteen and twenty four,' she informed me.

'What?'

I was genuinely amazed—not in a good way. It was no more than a few months since my last appointment and things had been stable then. All of a sudden, the pressures had gone up, either into the danger zone or to the edge of it.

'Your pressures are consistently too high,' she said.

Again, I was surprised, since they had been at an acceptable level for as long as I could remember.

'The trend is always up,' she explained, 'It is difficult to keep them fully under control.'

'What can be done?' I asked.

'We could adjust your eye drops,' she said, 'But you could have a trabeculoplasty.'

'What is that?'

'It is a new laser treatment that will provide a longer-term solution.'

'Not a cure?'

'No.'

I was beginning to realise what lay behind the dangerous door in the corridor. A new toy. And, wouldn't you know it, my pressures were up just at the moment that it had been installed!

But the treatment did sound worthwhile. Essentially, it works by using a laser to stimulate fluid drainage channels in the eye so that they work more effectively to expel excess aqueous humour. The bad news is that it does not obviate the need to take eye drops. It simply brings down the pressures and creates a means by which they can stay relatively low. It also only has a 66% success rate, so it is possible to go through it only to experience no benefits at all. If it works, it should keep on working for around two years. It is also easy to do—the doctor points a laser at the eye and blasts it in bursts in a rough circle pattern around the iris. No need for anaesthetics, no need to be admitted to hospital, no need for a lengthy recovery period. All sorted out in one visit to the clinic.

I talked to Karen about it next time I went up to Nottingham.

'A laser?' she asked.

'Yes, it's all a bit sci-fi,' I replied.

'How does it work?'

'Not sure.'

'But having a laser shone into your eyes—'

'Well, I suppose they know what they're doing.'

Karen was ever the pragmatist.

'Yes,' she said, 'it should be good.'

I was booked in for the treatment a couple of weeks later. When I spoke to Karen about it, I was unaccountably elated. It seemed like good news, a sort of semi-permanent solution that would guarantee me the chance to live my life normally. It didn't occur to me that, even if it worked, it would make no meaningful difference to my routines.

I returned to ACES for the treatment and sat in the waiting area. Light beams picked out by dust were luminescent fingers pointing at me through the arched window. I was not worried. As far as I could tell, there was only upside. If I were in the 33% for whom this was a futile exercise, I would still be where I was before. I would need to find some way to get the rampant pressures down, but there were ways to do that.

The dark spectre of an operation always lurked in the background. In some place at the back of my mind the thought was forming that maybe one lay in my future. The laser treatment was all well and good, but it was still another step on a downward sloping path. I had to admit that my glaucoma was getting worse and I was only in my forties. This should not have been happening for another twenty years at least.

I was called in to the laser room. It looked familiar. A chair for me, a chair for the doctor, a piece of machinery with a chin rest and various appendages. The Eastern European doctor was already there. She told me to sit down. I obeyed and placed my chin on the rest. I probably had dye put into my eyes, but I can't remember because I was now feeling unexpectedly nervous. I was about to have a laser fired at my eyes. A laser! I could only think of the machine as the Death Star and my eyeballs as Alderaan. What if she missed her target? What if the laser were accidentally on too high a setting? What if—

'Don't blink,' the doctor said.

My right eye saw the laser move into position. And then a red flash. Then another. Behind it, I could just make out the doctor in semi-silhouette lining up her gun like a sniper coolly zeroing in on her prey. Or maybe a gamer hunting pixilated pixies in some virtual fantasy world. Another flash. Oh, I thought, this hurts. Flash! It was painful. My eye felt like it was being repeatedly poked with a pointed stick. Flash! When would this end?

Flash! Flash! Flash!

Ouch!

'You can sit back now,' the doctor's clipped, emotionless voice said from somewhere in the dark.

I complied. Wow! That had not been remotely enjoyable. And there was still my other eye to do.

I lay my chin back on the rest like a French aristocrat kneeling before the guillotine.

A few minutes later, it was over. Both of my eyes felt pummeled and achey.

For the next couple of days, they were sore. Sensitivity to light was part of it: opening my lids in daylight caused me an initial stab of pain, followed by a persistent throbbing like that of a fresh bruise. I did not want to drive and so Karen came to visit me the following weekend. Getting dinner with her in a pizza restaurant in Peterborough, I was optimistic and positive about the procedure. As much as I was still having to take the drops, I could now anticipate a period of problem-free appointments.

When I went to ACES for a follow-up appointment, I was seen by a different doctor, one of those kindly old coves who are no longer in it for their careers.

'Let's have a look at your pressures, then, shall we?' he asked rhetorically.

I went through the usual process. The light shone in my eyes, looking into their depths, taking measurements.

'Oh yes,' the doctor said, as though celebrating a goal by his favourite football team, 'It's worked. Twelve and thirteen!'

'Thank God!' I said.

I had a two-year lease on those pressures. Those highs that had precipitated the procedure in the first place were gone—at least, for the time being.

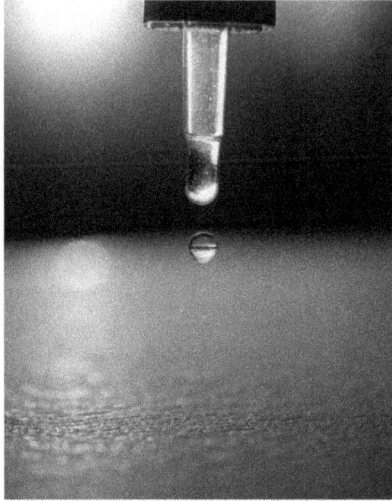

Chapter 7—One Drop at a Time

'YOU PUT YOUR drops in at the same time?'

'Yes.'

The pharmacist looked shocked. We were sitting in a consultation room (which was a glorified cupboard) in that pharmacy attached to the doctor's surgery in March. Since I had been taking the same medication for some considerable time, she had asked to have a chat to ensure that I was comfortable with it.

'That's not a good idea,' she told me.

'Oh, I assumed that they reinforced each other,' I explained.

'No,' she said, 'you should leave a few minutes between drops so that they can absorb properly into your eyes.'

'Thank you,' I said, 'I didn't know that.'

She seemed pleased that she had imparted that little piece of wisdom to me.

'Good,' she said, 'so that is one positive outcome from this meeting.'

This was true, although I had only gone into the pharmacy to pick up a prescription. As I left the room, the prescription was ready.

The assistant asked as she handed me a bag full of my drugs.

'Do you pay?'

'Twice over,' I said, 'once through my 40% marginal tax rate and once here.'

Her barely concealed scowl indicated that this quip had not gone down well.

I traipsed back to my car with my booty in my hand. These trips to March were becoming tedious now that I was based in Wisbech. The time had come to move my medical centre of gravity.

This would have advantages, but it would not be all good news. The best part was that the surgery with which I would register was on one of Wisbech's 'Brinks' and no more than a couple of hundred metres from where I lived. It also included a pharmacy that was open until 10pm. Less positively, it had an enormous number of patients on its books, which turned appointments into collectors' items. Also, like most Brink tenants, it occupied a renovated Georgian house. The only real waiting area was a corridor, the reception consisted of a hole-in-the-wall and there was nowhere to leave a car except a public car park across the road at the rear—and at certain times of the year, that was occupied by a travelling fair. Still, on balance, the advantages outweighed the disadvantages and I went in to complete the registration forms.

An issue was the length of time it would take for my application to be processed—potentially longer than my current collection of drops would last. In the event, I was able to get some new drops before my supply ran out, but it was a close-run thing: I was down to 'gusty puff of air' level with both. Shooting some cool wet medicine into my eyes felt like luxury after the drought that they had just gone through.

I started a regime of leaving around ten minutes in between applications of the two drops, in line with the pharmacist's advice. It quickly became a nuisance. Not only did it exacerbate the problem of forgetting whether I had applied the stuff at all, but it turned a relatively uncomplicated operation into one that took up a large chunk of the evening, not to mention the morning. I started to lapse into bad habits during the morning application. Soon enough, both the morning and evening applications had reverted to the old pattern. I reasoned that my pressures had been low for as long as I could remember, so I could not have been doing anything too wrong. Besides, I said to myself, the pharmacist was not a doctor! What did she know? It turned out—as I would discover after many another vicissitude—that the answer was 'quite a lot'.

I became starkly aware of the true negative of taking the drops whenever I went travelling. I had got into the habit of taking an annual road trip with a friend called Mike in one of the several sports cars that made up his—rather lavish—collection. The tradition began in 2001, in the pre-glaucoma days, with a long drive in a convertible Mercedes through France and Italy. It was revived over a decade later when we journeyed to Spain in a classic Porsche 911; the same car took us through Belgium, Switzerland and parts of Germany a year later. A Golf GTI was the mode of transport for journeys to Norway and Romania.

The nature of the trips meant that we would often be on the road until past the time at which I was meant to have applied the evening drops. This was solved once we stopped somewhere for the night, but I was often forced to medicate later than I should have been. Storage, too, was not a simple matter. I could not put the drops in my travel bag—that was in the car's boot, removing the option of applying the drops if we were still on the road at application time. So I carried the two bottles in my jacket pocket, which had the virtue of convenience, but, if the ambient temperature was high, they became alarmingly hot. Whether this affected the efficacy of their contents I could not say, but sometimes the drops were so warm that I would not feel them going into my eyes. On such occasions I tended to use far more than I needed to.

Over dinner somewhere in Germany during one of the trips, the matter came up in conversation.

'You have to take them how often?' Mike asked.

'Twice a day.'

'Fucking hell! It must be a pain in the arse.'

'It's okay. You get used to it.'

'Even so—'

'Everyone has something that they've got to put up with.'

'I suppose so. It's very sad, though. Maybe there'll be a cure at some point.'

'Maybe, but I suspect that I won't still be around to benefit from it.'

'You'd be surprised,' he said, 'Wait and see what AI can do—it's already changing things that we could hardly have dreamed of as kids.'

'Bionic eyes would be good!'

'It's not as far-fetched as you think.'

Professionally, he worked for a company that used technology to help clients with decision-making in healthcare—he knew what he was talking about.

Those trips carried us to some truly beautiful places. I stood at the edge of a lake in Norway, my gaze roving over the still water to the jagged snow-topped mountains beyond. I sipped coffee in a square made up of the confectionary-like baroque palaces of Bratislava. I took in the meandering craziness of the Transfagarasan Highway in Romania, moments before being driven around it accompanied by the exhilarated roar of a sports car's engine.

All of these images were records of a life lived—I hoped—to the full.

But they were almost all visual.

Even as I was experiencing them, imprinting them in my memory, I knew that the camera lens was faulty. I wanted to see. To really see. To see and record. Make those places a part of myself. And to do it while I still could. As I scanned the cityscape from the top of, say, a gothic tower in Valencia, I willed my eyes to work harder than they ever had, to take in every little nuance. The colours, the textures, the depths and the shallows, the light and the shade. I thought that my eyes were doing so. Later, much later, I was to find out that I was wrong and that there was more to the things I was looking at than I ever imagined.

For now, there was only so much that my eyes were prepared to do for me. Back home, the pressures were refusing to stay put. Only about a year after the laser treatment, a visit to ACES revealed that they were on the rise again, knocking on the door of the danger zone. I could barely conceal my disappointment.

'Can I do the laser thing again?' I asked.

Vile Jelly

The Eastern European doctor gave me a surprising answer.

'Yes.'

A possibility opened up to me: perhaps I could get my eyes zapped every couple of years and that would help to keep the pressures down— at least, for a while. Ever the killjoy, the doctor nixed this possibility.

'You can only do it twice and there's no guarantee that it will work the second time.'

I was puzzled.

'Why can I only do it twice?'

She gave an answer to the effect that it would only be effective twice and that any attempt to go through the procedure a third time would potentially do more harm than good.

Still, that meant that I had one roll of the dice left.

I was booked in and again went through the odd experience of my eyes becoming targets for some futuristic super gun. Walking back to my flat afterwards, my eyes hurting and hating the light, I wondered how it had ever come to this. Rarely have I been more acutely aware of that dividing line between the life before and after my glaucoma diagnosis.

Yet, I always questioned what I would give up in exchange for not having the disease: Karen? Certainly not! Glaucoma would be a small price to pay for her. My doctorate, then? Perhaps. It had not, at that time, made much difference to anything, but I did like having the title 'Dr'. Well then, my ability to write books? I had learned that I was going to get my first book published on that journey to Romania. I had been in the bar of one of the remote hotels in which Mike and I stayed when an email had come through. It had been a moment of great elation. Would I have given it up not to have glaucoma? I suppose that even getting one's name in print is not worth going blind for, but was I really going blind?

In the end, I would not have given up anything. It was purely a hypothetical in any case. There was nothing that I could give up.

I could split up with Karen, repudiate my doctorate, turn down my publishing contract, but it would all be in vain. The glaucoma would still be there. I would still be staring intently at statues, landscapes and the sleek curves of sports cars thinking to myself, 'I must do this now, while I still can...'

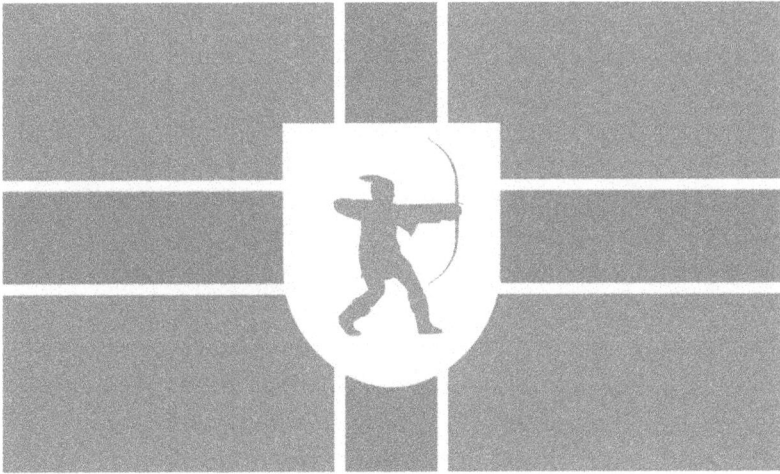

Chapter 8—New Starts

TOSH LEFT THE school.

It would be wrong to suggest that he acted on impulse. We had talked about the possibility at the Witch's and Café D'Light on numerous occasions. There were two drivers for his thinking, one was—

'German looks like it's going to be dropped from the curriculum.'

'Really?' I asked, surprised, 'But it's quite popular, isn't it?'

'We're not getting enough pupils. It's an option subject. Too few are choosing it.'

'You could teach French, couldn't you?'

The question was largely consolatory and rhetorical. He could teach French, but there were plenty of people already doing that—he was not needed. His job was in jeopardy, but that was not his real motive. His regular trips down south were taking their toll on his state of mind, not to mention finances. Luckily, Sharon—complete with family—had resolved to move up to Nottingham. One of the 'options' she and Tosh had discussed in the early days was his moving in with them, her moving to Wisbech having been mooted by Tosh and immediately dismissed.

He came in one day with his resignation letter in his pocket.

'Are you sure about this, mate?' I asked.

He was about to take that great step about which no teacher feels comfortable — quitting with no next job lined up. I was gutted at the prospect of it happening. Yes, he would be in Nottingham, a place in which I was spending an increasing amount of my time, but the Witch's, the chip shop and Café D'Light would all be visited no more—at least, not with Tosh.

He carried the letter around all morning undelivered. A decision was being tossed around in his head. In the event, his hand was forced. While in the photocopier room, he overheard someone say that the last day for resigning that year was upon us. What this meant was that, if Tosh did not act now, he would have to serve another term's notice before being able to leave. In practice, this would delay his moving in with Sharon by seven months. The revelation provoked in him a hasty march to the headmaster's office. It was a moment of bravado like that of the Woody Allen character in *Manhattan* storming out of his TV gig for good.

We shared a slightly dubious drink at the Witch's after work. Nominally a celebration, it was actually an informal therapy session for a man who had just done something that went against his nature. Tosh was, after all, the person who had told me that he hated change and would happily have spent his entire career at the college at which he had previously worked had he not been made redundant. This is not to imply that he lacked ambition, but, when making major decisions, his head usually beat his heart.

As a boy, he had left a school in Bradford, at which he had been happy, for the more academically rigorous environment of its counterpart in Worcester. When contemplating University, he had weighed up whether to go to Cambridge, Liverpool—which would have allowed him to get a season ticket for his beloved hometown football team—or to follow his then girlfriend to France, where he could have studied German at the University of Rennes. Cambridge was the smart choice. In fact, his recent resignation had been the only occasion upon which he had given way to what his heart wanted. Hence, he was more than a little nervous about what he had done. But he expressed no regret—which he has always rejected as a useless emotion.

'It's the best thing I've done,' he said, 'Start a new life. Be with someone.'

'Exactly,' I said, supportively, 'The worst thing that can happen is that you might have to do a bit of supply teaching for a while. You've got plenty of ways to earn a few quid.'

In truth, I envied him. I had long wished that I could give up the daily drudgery of working for someone else and just do my own thing. I was not afraid to take the plunge. I had quit with no job to go to before— I was to again, although not in such an atmosphere of risk. I had also completely changed careers. At that moment, I had similar pull factors to those which were working on Tosh: Karen was desperate for me to move to Nottingham to be with her. But the weight of the Wisbech flat's mortgage was holding me down. Some sort of settlement around that was needed if I were to even contemplate a life without a steady income.

But a seed had been planted. Tosh's last day was the end of the summer term. As was typical of him, there was not much of a gap between one stage of his life and the next. There was no fanfare, no last hurrah, no victory lap, no party. He finished on a Friday afternoon and was on the X1 before there was time to say, 'cheerio.' In an obscure kind of way, I felt that I, too, was on borrowed time. My other good friend—and member of my department—Emma, with whom I had worked at two schools over the course of sixteen years, had also recently departed for a job in Surrey. The sense of an era coming to an end was overwhelming. It would not be long, I felt, before I followed them out of the door.

It happened sooner than expected.

In August, the external exam results were published. As much as I always wanted the world to be astounded at what we, the English Department, had achieved with our pupils, those pupils were, in the end, kids and they achieved what they were bound to achieve. Some did better than expected, some did worse. Most reached their predicted level. There was no way to alter that through my own deeds. It did not matter what I accomplished personally. It did not matter what talents I may or may not have possessed, or how good a teacher I was. I could not break the ceiling of my pupils' capabilities. As I walked away from the school on results day, I felt that I had spent long enough trying and that it was someone else's turn. It was time to focus on what I could – or could not – achieve for myself. At the start of term, I handed in my own letter.

It was a Friday. That evening, I drove up to visit Karen. She was delighted to see me and said that we should go for dinner in town to celebrate my momentous decision. Curiously, she did not want to drive, as was habitual, but to walk from her house to the restaurant. This was not too much of an imposition—the distance was not huge—but it was unprecedented. I went along with it. The weather was mild and it was still the time of year when daylight lasted until well into the evening. I soon realised what she was up to. On entering the restaurant, I saw a reserved table by the window in the middle of which was an ice bucket containing a bottle of Prosecco. If I had had any doubts about the wisdom of my leaving the school, she did not.

We sat down and I poured us each a glass of the wine. I had that feeling that I always get when I cut the ties to something that I perceive to be holding me back. One of possibility. Excitement. I had been at the school for just under ten years—it would be ten years by the time I left—but now the future was no longer so determined. I could change direction, do something new, go anywhere I liked...

Provided, of course, that I could ensure a regular supply of eye drops. And I would obviously need access to a hospital or clinic. I couldn't do absolutely anything, then, but I could do most things. As long as whatever it was paid enough for me to be able to afford medical care if I happened to be in a foreign country. But, apart from all that, I was free to do whatever I wanted! As long as my vision did not deteriorate to the point at which I would need an operation...

As we sipped our drinks, Karen and I talked about plans and possibilities. We took it for granted that we would be together. Karen was typically bullish. She had been self-employed for years, so harboured no fears at all about our chances of moving on successfully.

One possibility we talked about was Malaysia. It happened that, an advert had recently appeared requesting applications for posts on a

World Bank Funded scheme to teach at the branch campus of a British university in that distant country. The students would not be Malaysians, but college teachers from Bangladesh. The idea was to teach them educational leadership skills and turn them into motors of reform in the colleges in which they worked. It was run by a university professor who I knew.

'Do you think I should go for it?' I asked.

Karen did not look all that keen.

'It's a long way away,' she said.

'Yes, but I have always talked about working abroad. This could be my chance.'

I refreshed our glasses.

'What about your eyes?'

'I would get medical insurance,' I said.

'But what are their hospitals like?"

That I did not know. And she was right to be concerned. If Malaysia's clinics and hospitals were not up to providing the kind of eye care that I had been used to, moving there would be a huge gamble. But I remembered the words of the first glaucoma doctor I had seen in March. He had been in favour of the idea of my seeking jobs abroad.

'I think I should go for it,' I said.

Karen said nothing. She sipped her wine and gave a weak half-smile.

I followed my instincts and had an online interview. An emailed offer duly came through from that professor. Karen and I were about to go into a theatre on the evening that I received it to see a comedy show that I had first caught at the Edinburgh Festival the year before. It failed to raise so much as a titter from her. I could sense that something was wrong.

'How did you enjoy that?' I asked her afterwards.

'I didn't really take it in,' she said.

'What's wrong?' I pressed.

'It's alright,' she said.

She was subdued for the remainder of the evening. The next morning, I raised it with her. We were sitting at the wooden breakfast bar in her kitchen. The atmosphere was sombre.

'It's because of this job offer, isn't it?' I said.

She did not speak, but I could tell. Neither of us had been that young when we met. Whether our relationship was anything as dramatic as a 'last chance for love' I would doubt, but Karen had invested six years of her life in it at a time when six years could not lightly be cast aside.

Six years! That hit me. Six years: a long time. How much more certain did I need to be? In a moment of supreme inspiration, I came to a decision.

'Look,' I said, 'If you want me to reassure you that I have got every intention of coming back, why don't we get married?'

Her jaw dropped like something out of a cartoon.

'What?' she asked.

'Let's get married,' I repeated, 'Then you will know that I am not going to disappear to Asia and not return.'

No response came there and then.

Instead, I was summoned back the following Friday 'to talk about stuff.'

In the muted lighting of Karen's kitchen, we sat again at the breakfast bar with a glass each of white wine.

'This is what I have decided,' she began, 'We get married, then you go to Malaysia for a year and I will come out every few months to visit as your wife.'

'Why don't you just come out to live with me?' I suggested.

'You know I have to look after my mum,' she said, 'I can't abandon her; I just can't.'

This was fair enough. Her mum lived nearby and was not in good health. She was getting on in age—to say the least. Karen was her only real carer.

'For a year?' I weighed it up. My job offer was for two years initially, which, in all honesty, was the more likely duration of my time away. Still, everything else about this was good.

'Yes, okay,' I said, 'Let's do it. Let's get married.'

'Agreed.'

'Well, I suppose that we'd better go out and celebrate.'

While this arrangement was exciting in many ways, it would not be true to say that everything suddenly fell into place. For a start, I had not been sent a formal job offer as such. An email from someone who happened to be at the interview was a slender hook on which to hang my life. At that precise moment, I was in the position of having resigned from one job without having definitely secured another. Even if the Malaysia job was real—I had no reason to suppose that it was not—I did not know when it was due to start. It could be soon, it could be in several months. Karen and I decided, then, to get married as soon as was practicable.

In such circumstances, Karen comes very much into her own. Few people I know are better at making things happen. Almost immediately, we were on our way out of Nottingham to a Hall in the country that she wanted to book for the ceremony and the reception.

It was nice. A little scruffy and rundown for sure, but it had character. The bar was an atmospheric little room, filled with overstuffed leather sofas. A French window opened on to a well-kept garden. There was also a conservatory that we were told was where the ceremony would take place. We booked it, only to read some reviews later that were less than complimentary. Never mind, we thought, it fitted our requirements and was available at short notice. A ten-week countdown until the chosen date at the end of January began.

While all that was going on, Tosh's 50th birthday party happened. It was Bonfire Night—November 5th—2016 when Karen and I, as well as a whole lot of Tosh and Sharon's friends and mutual friends, assembled at Arnold Liberal Club in Nottingham for the event.

Karen and I were among the few more-or-less fully sighted people there. One of Tosh's (and my) former colleagues had also made the trek up from Wisbech. Plenty of guide dogs were present. They were extremely well-behaved, sitting quietly under tables or alongside chairs and banquettes. Their training came through strongly.

I spent much of the evening talking to Tosh's internet radio-operating friends.

'How is it going?' I asked.

'Well, it's going,' one, a 'total', replied with some sarcasm.

I pressed.

'Oh, not too well?'

He sighed.

'It's okay, but it takes a while to build. There's a lot of internet radio stations out there. We've set some ambitious listener targets.'

'What are you getting at the moment?'

'We got up to thirty-five last Sunday.'

I was impressed.

'Thirty-five—what?—hundred? That's all right!'

He laughed mirthlessly.

'No. Thirty-five listeners.'

'Oh…'

I now understood why my requests were always played. There were probably times when Tosh and I were the only people tuning in.

Shortly after everyone had eaten, Tosh called the room to order so that he could make a short speech.

'Thank you for coming,' he began, 'I hope that you are enjoying the evening. I know I am! Time is getting on. It feels strange to be fifty. Another step on the road to the Big Sleep, but many happy returns, I hope. But I am guilty of some duplicity because this is not just a birthday party. As you know, I have been in a relationship with Sharon and a couple of weeks ago, she agreed to become my wife. So this is, in fact, a joint birthday and engagement celebration.'

At this news, a gasp of surprise passed around the room, to be followed by congratulatory applause. There was a smile on every face. I was not among those who gasped. I had suspected that a gathering this large was unlikely to be just for an annual event that Tosh treats with as much disdain as I do.

'Thank you,' Tosh went on, 'The night's not over yet. We've got plenty of music to come and the buffet is not finished!'

One of Tosh's VI radio DJ friends got the turntables going and the party turned into a disco. I went over to Tosh.

'Congratulations!' I said.

'Thanks, mate,' he replied, 'And we talked about this some months ago, just so you know.'

It was a strange and rather confrontational remark, but I fully understood it. He was indicating that his decision to marry was not influenced by anything that Karen and I had done. He need not have worried. I knew. I had known since his first face-to-face meeting with Sharon.

'It's all right,' I said, putting my arm around his shoulder. 'I get it.'

The dance floor filled up. At one point, Karen, Tosh, his newly announced fiancée and I jigged around in a rather middle-aged way. Two engaged couples together, enjoying some eighties pop song or other. Our former colleague and his wife joined in. The guide dogs watched insouciantly from the side lines.

Tosh had set a date some fourteen months hence. Karen and I had a more urgent deadline.

Quite without planning it, we introduced something of an ocular theme into the musical choices for our wedding. At some point, we had decided that *Teardrop* by Massive Attack was 'our song'. Why was lost in the cascading memories of our early relationship—it was probably just a rare song that we both loved—but it had become something of a leitmotif of our time together.

Lyrically, it deals with eyes quite a lot. Obviously, eyes are where teardrops originate but also included is the line: 'Water is my eye / Most faithful mirror'. While the emphasis is on the eye as a mechanism, it is a reminder of the centrality of eyes in the human experience. We decided not only to make *Teardrop* our first-dance song, but we would use an instrumental version of it by the jazz combo The Robert Mitchell 3io to accompany Karen's walk down the 'aisle'.

Playlisting aside, there were numerous other tasks to accomplish, although everything was much less trouble than when I had first married in the 90s. I organised the rings and my outfit—sort of. I was keen on a Paul Smith suit. Karen preferred Hugo Boss. I got Hugo Boss.

I also asked Tosh to sing a song at the ceremony. Both Karen and I wanted to make the day as much fun as possible and Tosh possessed a famously excellent singing voice. At first, Karen was dubious. She tried to edge Tosh's contribution towards being more like a traditional reading, but I insisted. The plan was to provide a backing track to which he could add the vocals. I also suggested that it be in German, which caused further trepidation for Karen. We chose a song called, *Du Bist Das Licht*, originally by one Gregor Meyle. In another inadvertent nod to eyesight, the title means *You Are The Light*.

The wedding went off well, on the whole. Tosh's recorded backing cut out at one point, but he, ever the trouper, kept going and got through it. Almost everyone present later averred that his moment had been the undisputed highlight of the day. The band that we booked, however, were more of a curate's egg. They could not play *Teardrop*, so, despite our handing over a chunky fee for their services, Karen and I had our first dance to a CD. Worse even than that, Wolverhampton Wanderers beat Liverpool in the Premier League! My mother's husband was a 'Wolves' fan. He rather gleefully reminded Tosh of the result as frequently as possible.

Karen and I stayed in the hall that night. We were the only guests. The next morning, we had breakfast, headed back to Nottingham and had a cup of tea in a vegan café. Then I went back to Wisbech. I was to remain there for three months until my contract with the school ended. But, once it had, Karen and I only ended up living together for a short time because the HR department from the Malaysian University finally got in touch.

I was due to start work in July.

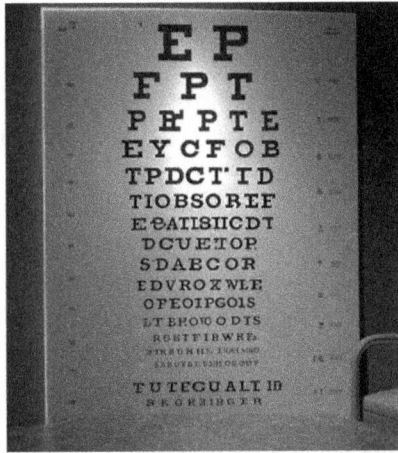

Chapter 9—A Glaucomatous Englishman Abroad

ROAD TRIPS ARE one thing, but the real trouble around eye drops comes with flying—especially long haul flying. I was accustomed to applying the drops in the morning and then twelve hours later in the evening. That was all very well, but what about when twelve hours is no longer twelve hours? What about when twelve hours is twenty hours? Or twenty-four hours? I was heading to Malaysia, a twelve-to-fourteen-hour flight if taken direct—and there were not really any direct flights to speak of from the UK.

My journey began in Birmingham in the late afternoon with a seven-hour flight to Dubai, the time zone for which put it three hours ahead of the UK, followed by another seven-to-eight-hour flight to Kuala Lumpur, which was four further hours ahead. I arrived in Malaysia in the late afternoon of the following day, having been travelling for fifteen hours, but with twenty-four hours or so having passed in the real world—or whichever world was real at any given moment during my flight. When, therefore, was I to put my eye drops in? And, once I was into a whole new routine, how would that play out with what I had previously been doing? Would the interval between my last application of the drops in the UK and my first in Malaysia be too long or too short?

This may all seem difficult, but it was as nothing compared to the problems that I would encounter when the phrase 'preservative free' entered my life some months later. That was the point at which flying became a particular bugbear...

Prior to leaving the UK, I was obliged to have a medical examination and a drug test. The latter was fairly straightforward—it was to establish whether I was a user of any illegal substances. Since I never had been, I did not fear it. The more general medical examination was probably to ensure that I would not be a strain on Malaysia's public services. Both proved to be much harder to arrange than I expected.

I tried my GP, only to discover that getting a medical examination on the NHS was unlikely bordering on impossible. Not to worry! I had, for some years, been paying an insurance company for private medical cover. They, I was sure, would do the examination. I called them.

'I would like to arrange a medical examination, please,' I said to the man at the other end of the line.

'For what purpose?'

I explained that I had a job in Malaysia and I was required to provide a medical certificate before taking it up.

'Oh yes,' the man said, 'We don't do those.'

'What?'

'We don't do medical checks for jobs.'

'Why not?'

'We just don't.'

This was not the first time I had had a version of this conversation. I had previously enquired about a contribution to the cost of my more conventional eye tests. Nothing doing there either. I was a little exasperated.

'So what do you do?' I asked.

'We provide you with cover for any medical needs that you have.'

'Except my eyes,' I said, 'which happens to be the only thing that's wrong with me.'

This was true. When I had taken out the plan, my glaucoma had been specifically excluded as a 'pre-existing condition'.

'I'm sorry to disappoint you,' the man said superciliously.

'So, to be clear, I'm paying you sixty pounds a month for nothing.'

'We cover your medical needs.'

'Every time I've asked you to cover a medical need, you've said "no", so I come back to what I said—you are taking my money every month for nothing at all.'

'Thank you for calling,' he said.

The line went dead.

A big advantage of moving abroad would be cancelling that 'insurance' and saving myself what was effectively a voluntary tax.

At that precise moment, though, I was in a bind. How exactly was I going to get an examination done? I called the British branch of the University in question. They were somewhat bemused. This had never really come up before. They had not heard of anyone experiencing difficulties with getting a doctor to do a quick once-over. They suggested using the University's own clinic. I paid it a visit. Sorry, no: have you thought about going to your own GP?

What to do?

I called a private clinic in Nottingham. Yes, they could do both the drug test and the medical examination—for a hefty price. I had no real choice. I booked myself in.

The place was what I always imagined a private clinic might look like: not so much a doctor's surgery as the office of a property magnate. The doctor was dressed in a suit that looked like it cost more than the Royal Navy. The receptionist who let me in was a stark contrast to her frazzled and overworked counterpart at my GP's surgery. She greeted me with a solicitous air and the offer of a coffee. I declined with thanks and sat in a leather armchair in the waiting room. I was the only patient there. That was another difference from the clinic in Wisbech, which was permanently busy. This was quiet, calming.

For the drug test, I provided a urine sample into which various lollipop stick like probes were dipped before being subjected to some kind of analysis. As I expected, I came up clean on every count.

The main medical examination was the standard thing. I am happy to say that there was no squeezing of my balls accompanied with a cough, but lights were shone into my ears, my weight was recorded, my height checked. I was asked to balance on one leg.

When it came to my eyes, a crisis that I knew was coming was reached.

'Do you have any eye conditions?' the doctor asked, no doubt expecting a bland answer.

'I'm pretty short-sighted,' I said, 'and I have glaucoma.'

'Oh,' he said, 'Okay. Do you have to take medication?'

'Eye drops. Twice a day.'

He realised that this might be a dealbreaker for the job, so helpfully put onto the form that I had 'slight' glaucoma. There was no way for him to check the severity of the disease, but he was prepared to do me a favour. My vision test was not so promising. Without glasses, I could barely see the board, much less any letters on it. No matter. The doctor wrote that I needed to wear glasses to correct my vision. He wrote at some length, the better to bury the detail about the glaucoma.

Several hundred pounds the poorer, I went away with the pieces of paper that I needed. But that was not the end of my medical preparations for Malaysia. I still needed to get some vaccinations. I was not really sure what to expect from the country in which I would soon be an immigrant. My experience of East Asia was limited: I had visited Hong Kong a couple of times, but that was all. Some of my friends seemed to think that Malaysia would be a second North Korea. Everyone averred that I had better get some vaccinations, since I would be at risk from all manner of tropical diseases that would kill an ill-prepared Northern European within seconds of his arrival.

I knew that I needed a 'jab' for Hepatitis (which I was unaware had a whole alphabet's worth of variations) but was not sure about any others. I went back to the University clinic. They breezily told me that they had no hepatitis vaccine. In a spooky premonition of my future with out-of-stock eye drops, ringing around a number of clinics returned the same result: there was no vaccine available. I tried my GP. They had some! Appointments were at a premium, but I managed to land one. It was a little too close to my leaving date for comfort, but I would still be fine, unless something went drastically wrong.

The appointment was in Wisbech. By now, I was living in Nottingham. But that was all right. Getting from one to the other would only take an hour and a half or so. They were connected by the A1, which was never congested. I set off in the morning. I gave myself plenty of time. So much so, that I anticipated having to wait for a while in Café D'Light before going into the surgery.

For the first time ever in my experience, the A1 was gridlocked with traffic. As the MX5 moved forward centimetres at a time, I incessantly checked the clock. Okay. Not in trouble yet. I'm okay. Time passed. So there won't be any café time. That's not a problem. I would just get the vaccines over with and head home. More time passed. If the way were clear on the other side of Peterborough, I could still make it. I used the Bluetooth kit that I had had installed to call the surgery and let them know I might be late. No one answered. The time of the appointment came and went.

The road cleared. Predictably, the delay seemed to have been caused by nothing at all. By the time I had reached Wisbech, parked the car and rushed into the clinic, my appointment was nearly two hours in the past. I asked the receptionist if I could re-arrange it for later in the day. That, I was told, could not be done under any circumstances. The next available slot was not until after I was due to have flown to Malaysia.

I called another costly private clinic in Nottingham. They had some of the vaccine. But, they asked, what did I need it for? I am going to work in Malaysia, I said. Oh no, they said, you will need more than just one jab. You will need vaccinations against two strains of hepatitis, rabies, malaria, typhoid, diphtheria, cholera and something called Japanese Encephalitis. Do I actually need this last one? I asked. Oh yes, they said, it is rare, for sure, but if you catch it—it is borne by a particular type of fly—your brain will swell up and you will die horribly. Okay, I said, I'd better have them all. Great, they said, that will be six hundred pounds please.

Another problem was that the hepatitis vaccines were courses, rather than single shots. Because I was so close to my leaving date, I was only able to get the first of the three that I needed. This more-or-less compelled me to fly home for Christmas so that I could get the second shot, which, even so, would be late. In the event, it proved to be quite a propitious return for my eyes as well. I was told all of this while sitting in the plush office of a private clinic by a well-educated and wealthy-looking young male doctor who spent most of my consultation moaning about the British Empire.

Given how primitive I was being led to believe Malaysia to be, a concomitant worry was whether the care that my eyes needed would even be available out there. If it proved difficult to get treatment, I would have to cut my stay short. I hedged my bets by going to the clinic in Wisbech and asking for an over-supply of eye drops. It was the first time that I had ever met 'my' doctor. I explained that I was going out to Malaysia and that, although medical insurance was part of my package, I was not sure how long it would take me to set up regular eyecare. Could I, therefore, have three months' worth of drops to keep me covered while I investigated the medical possibilities? This, I was told, would not be a problem. A prescription was written and I went into the practice's own pharmacy, which was homely in feel, and came away with a large bag of small bottles to stow in my luggage.

Medical examinations complete, vaccines sort-of done and my eyes catered for, there was nothing left to do but fly out and get on with it. It was quite a leap in the dark. I knew nothing about the University I was going to and had little idea about where I would live beyond having been assured that a 'bungalow' on campus was available for the first two weeks.

The day before my flight, Karen and I went for lunch at a restaurant called La Rock. It was an upmarket establishment, one of those—of which there are many—that inexplicably lack a Michelin star despite their excellence. Afterwards, we had a stroll along the canal opposite. It somehow did not seem real that I would be disappearing for so long so soon. We chatted as though nothing out of the ordinary was happening.

That last meal had barely been digested when we headed for Birmingham Airport. My 'big stash' of eye drops was inside my check-in bag. In the pockets of my jacket, I carried the bottles that I would use during the flight. Karen and I had a coffee together in a cafe this side of Security. She seemed sad but was buoyed by the thought that she would be visiting in September and that I would be home for a couple of weeks over Christmas. We would not be apart for too long. I was only to discover how important this whole thing was to her when I first met my boss in Malaysia, who told me that she had received several calls from Karen asking about my timetable so that visits could be pre-scheduled. On the one hand, I was angry, but, on the other, it was touching that my wife was so concerned to ensure that we would have opportunities to spend time together.

Back at Birmingham Airport, Karen and I had a final hug and kiss and I went in to start what would be a new life, or, at least, a new phase of life.

My next eye drop application was due to be during the first leg to Dubai. I placed my jacket in an overhead locker. Unfortunately, I did not have an aisle seat. I would have to ask the person sitting next to me to let me out when I needed to take the drops. That would be annoying, but, as it happened, when the moment came, we were experiencing turbulence: I was not permitted to leave my seat at all. I prayed for the plane to stop bouncing around. Eventually, it did and I put the eye drops in as best as I could while standing in the aisle. One, then, immediately, the other—I had long since jettisoned the March pharmacist's advice on the grounds of its being 'a pain in the arse'.

Malaysia defied the warnings of my friends by being modern, beautiful and tolerant. It was a wonderful place to live. Once my stay in the bungalow was over, I moved into a room in a compound close to the University. Basically a student hall of residence, it was not the most luxurious of homes, but it served a purpose and I remained there for the entirety of my time in the country. It had the considerable advantage of containing a number of restaurants, snack bars and the shop which was to become my lifeline during periods when the country closed down for one or other of its frequent public holidays. There was also a bar, an antidote to the University's campus being 'dry'.

Some months after moving in, I spent an evening in that bar with David, a colleague from the Psychology Department who specialised in illnesses around vision and eyesight. We sat with pints of Tiger Beer at high tables on the decking that overlooked a landscaped tropical garden.

The conversation meandered around to the subject of my glaucoma.

'Wow,' David said. 'So you have to take medication?'

I described the eye drops.

'Will it get worse?'

'I suppose it will,' I admitted.

'So you may have really serious eyesight loss in later life.'

Yes. Probably. He had astutely keyed into my greatest fear, that the retirement to which I had been looking forward for decades was slipping away from me. The adventures that I had anticipated having once work was no longer a part of my life, the worlds that I had thought to explore—perhaps, after all, I would have nothing to do but mope around a house that I could barely see, if I could see it at all. It felt like the most unkindest cut of all.

Not long after I arrived, new hires were given a presentation by the company that provided our medical insurance. The big news for me was that the cost of prescriptions would be covered. No more exorbitant charges! Well, maybe…as I was to discover, it did not work out quite like that. For a start, there was a qualifying period; for several months, I would be paying full price. Plus, medical treatment would end up being by no means as completely free of charge as promised.

But, for a while, all that was academic. My supply of eye drops from home kept me going. I was not in a hurry to reach its end, since I imagined that finding replacements might prove difficult. I fantasised that the drops that I had would last until I returned to the UK at Christmas, but my sense of realism was less hopeful.

Soon enough, the drops began to run low. It was, moreover, some months since my last checkup. I discussed this with Karen over Facebook Messenger. Perhaps I could visit the clinic while I was home? If so, I would only need to secure a source of the drops in Malaysia temporarily.

Accomplishing that turned out to be nowhere near as complicated as it was in the UK. The drops could be picked up from any pharmacist with a single prescription. They were relatively cheap. I paid a visit to the University doctor, who, handily, occupied an office just along from that of the project on which I was working. She, like the majority of doctors with whom I would come into contact while out there, was

Malaysian Indian. I sat at the end of her desk and explained my situation.

'You've got glaucoma?' she said in the matter-of-fact tone of a professional who knew all the implications and was already formulating a strategy.

'Yes,' I said.

'Do you want a prescription?'

'Yes, please.'

It was that simple. She wrote me a note that I could take to any pharmacy. Job done!

Or, it would have been if money had not quickly become something of a problem. Opening a bank account was not the simplest of operations. To do it, I needed a letter from my employer, not to mention my passport. Unfortunately, I could not obtain the letter until my 'Malaysia Pass'—essentially a work permit—had been glued into my passport, which could take a couple of months. The silver lining, if it can be called that, was that I didn't get paid during that period in any case. I had been told to bring enough cash from the UK to last me for around sixty days, which was a fair estimate of how long the wheels of bureaucracy would take to turn. I took six hundred pounds, reckoning that ten a day would be plenty. But, once I had paid the rent for my room, my coffers were severely depleted. I watched with horror as my pile of Malaysian ringgits grew ever smaller, despite my living a relatively frugal life. It was a question of which would run out first, my eye drops or my money.

I was down to about my last thirty pounds when, suddenly, I got the letter, opened my bank account and watched with some satisfaction as two months' salary was deposited into it in one go. It was late August. Three months of freewheeling with the drops that I was on before seeing a doctor back in the UK was not, I considered, going to be too much of a problem. For that interval I became a regular customer of a pharmacy next to the local branch of the supermarket Tesco.

Just before Christmas, Karen picked me up from Birmingham Airport. I was long overdue an eye examination. I had assumed that I could secure an appointment with ACES—where I was still registered. I had reckoned without the holidays. The place was closed up. A few calls got me into a clinic that was being held in the town of Whittlesey, which lay between March and Peterborough. The road to it passed through that old familiar flat landscape that afforded no cover to any object. From a distance, cars looked like they were driving straight through plowed fields.

The clinic was held in a building that was not bespoke, but, like its equivalent in March, was multi-purpose. My appointment was in the late afternoon at that time of year when darkness descends early. The place was eerily quiet. I was examined by a doctor I had never seen before, a no-nonsense type who looked like he ran iron man marathons for fun. My pressures were quite good. I took a fields test.

'Everything seems to be stable at the moment,' the doctor told me.

'Good,' I said, with an air of relief.

'We will give you a different type of fields test from now on, though,' he went on.

'Oh,' I said, puzzled.

'You don't seem to be that good at this one.'

'I don't really enjoy it,' I confessed.

'No one does,' he said, 'So we'll give you a simpler type of test. How often do you have an examination?"

'On average,' I calculated, 'every six months or so.'

'We'll change that to every four months,' he said, 'Just so that we can monitor your progress more closely.'

This all sounded out of sync with the news that my pressures were low and everything was basically all right. I was obviously missing something.

'Okay,' I began, 'but—'

'You must get an appointment every four months,' he said to me stridently, like a teacher telling off a naughty kid.

A couple of days later, I met Tosh for a drink in Nottingham. We sat in the street outside our favourite town centre pub. I had a boring lager and Tosh ordered a real ale that went under the name of Goose Gobbler, or something similar. The evening was cool, but we passed an enjoyable couple of hours watching people pass by. I wondered what challenges and struggles they were hiding under the self-absorption and air of urgency that they exhibited as they went from who-knew-where to who-knew-where. Tosh's wedding was scheduled to take place a month later. I would not be in the country for it, but Karen was on the guest list. One of Tosh's VI friends was tasked with being best man.

'How are the preparations going?' I asked.

'Very well, mate,' he said, 'Not that I'm doing much. I'm about as much use as an ashtray on a motorbike when it comes to this sort of thing.'

He sipped his real ale. I drew on my lager.

'How's Malaysia?' he asked.

'It's good, mate. I haven't done a lot yet, to be honest. We're still waiting for our first cohort of trainees to turn up.'

'Still?' He sounded amazed, 'You've been out there for nearly six months!'

'Well, we have had some trainees. Just not any that I am down to teach yet. I think that we have had some administrative teething troubles.'

'Fucking tyrannosaurus teeth by the sounds of it.'

I changed the subject.

'You know, everyone out in Malaysia's obsessed with Manchester United.'

'Really?'

'Yes. It is nearly impossible to rest your eyes on any scene without seeing some guy wearing a Man U replica shirt.'

'Christ! Sounds like somewhere for me to avoid,' he said.

For context, it should be said that, of Tosh's many pet peeves, close to the top of the list was Manchester United football club. While his dislike of them did not reach the mouth-frothing levels of hatred expressed by other people of my acquaintance, it was still the case that few things cheered him up quite as much as a Manchester United defeat.

'Listen, mate,' he said, a little nervously, 'About the wedding. We're sorry you can't be there, but we'd like you to do something like the thing that I did for you...'

'Not sure my voice is strong enough to reach from South East Asia, mate!'

'No, I know. But we were thinking that maybe you could write something—like a poem or something that we could get someone, Jane maybe, to read out.'

Jane was our former colleague and mutual friend. She enjoyed a position of unusual esteem for both of us. She had been at Oxford at the same time as me. We had not known each other then, but we had had acquaintances in common and I had heard her play with various student orchestras, without, obviously, knowing who she was.

'I would be honoured!' I said, more than a little moved by the request.

I started to write as soon as I parted from him. I knew that a Shakespearean sonnet would be the best model. As for a theme? One seemed obvious. The words flowed as though writing themselves.

If love is light, then little love have I,
With eyes like marbles, mere plugs in my skull,
The sun is lost to me, the stars are dull,
No sparks fill the sky when meteors fly.

But love is not in the gift of some high,
Aloof goddess with the wings of a gull:
Its truth lies deep in a heart that is full
Of the tender beats behind a soft sigh.

Therefore, love, let us take this golden band
That catches a light which we cannot see
And use it to join, in love, hand and hand.

Though we are blind, all the poets agree
That Love is, too, and they well understand
That we go by touch, not sights quickly scanned.

I suppose I thought that the imagined speaker was Tosh himself. But it could also have been my own future self. I emailed it to Tosh and awaited a response. He declared himself delighted.

The Whittlesey doctor's rather urgent words underlined the need for me to sort out some eye care in Malaysia. Upon my return, I went back to the University doctor for advice.

'What I need,' I told her, 'is access to a clinic or hospital that I can get some appointments with; I am supposed to get an examination every four months.'

She recommended two possibilities. One was a private Hospital called Taipan in KL—Kuala Lumpur. The other was a name I forget, although it was a specialist eye hospital. For some reason, I decided on Taipan. I called them and arranged an appointment.

The University and, therefore, my accommodation, were not actually in KL, but a town some distance away. The simplest way to get into the city was the train service known as the MRT. The nearest station was in a suburb called Kajang, which was some miles from where I was living. The best way to get to Kajang Station was to take a Grab - a local version of an Uber. At the other end, in KL, it was necessary to take another Grab from the MRT station—KL Sentral was best—to the hospital. This all took around an hour. I have gone into detail because it will become important later.

As I climbed out of a Grab on my first visit to the hospital, I could immediately see why Malaysia enjoys a reputation for excellent healthcare—and why all those cautions that people issued me with before I came were so wrong-headed; indeed, almost bigoted.

The hospital was located in one of the city's more upmarket areas and looked less like an institution devoted to curing people of illnesses than a five-star hotel. A large branch of Starbucks occupied a portion of the ground floor, but it was only one of a number of similar outlets. A huge concrete portico led to the main reception area, which was dotted here and there with armchairs and couches. The plush welcome desk was staffed by a couple of young women in smart corporate livery. I asked one of them where the eye clinic was to be found. She directed me to a corridor nearby.

A modest door took me into the clinic. I was directed to sit in a leather-upholstered armchair and wait to be called. After a while, a nurse appeared and said loudly: 'Mr Adrian!

Vile Jelly

One of the more endearing aspects of life in Malaysia is the way that first and second names are transposed. I was always 'Dr Adrian' at work, not 'Dr Jarvis'.

I followed the nurse into an examination room, in which she gave me the L-shaped device that I could use to cover my eyes in turn while the other was being used to pick out letters on a chart in front of me. As always, my right eye comfortably won that competition.

Another short wait, then I met the doctor, a short Malaysian Indian woman in early middle age with a serious professional air, who was not above some genteel chat to put her patients at ease. She asked me how I was feeling and I told her 'fine'—because that's what English people do. I was to get to know her quite well over the next three and a half years.

She took my pressures, which were not bad, but not quite as low as they had been when I had visited the clinic in Whittlesey. She pronounced herself satisfied for now and prescribed me a repeat of my usual eye drops. One area that did cause her some concern was the dryness of my eyes. I had been told something similar by opticians before now.

I picked up my prescription note at the reception. I hardly even listened to the reassurance that there was 'nothing to pay'. I took the note to the hospital's in-house pharmacy. It belied everywhere else in that building by being sparse, businesslike, not somewhere to linger. Behind the counter there was nothing to see other than closed drawers and locked cabinets. A lone assistant stood at one end. She took my note.

'We will have to get a GL,' she said.

'What's that?' I asked.

'A guarantee letter,' she explained, 'from the insurance company to say that they will cover the cost of the medicines.'

'Oh, right,' I said, 'How long will that take?'

'About an hour. We can call you when it has come through.'

I left my mobile number and headed for Starbucks. I had assumed that the insurance would kick in without need for further action on my part. But it was not too much of a problem. The hospital was so replete with facilities that spending more time there was a positive joy. The Starbucks was tastefully lit and occupied by people working on laptops or talking on mobile phones. I sipped an Americano waiting for the pharmacy to get in touch. In much less than an hour, they did and I went back to pick up my medicines.

Tosh and I were in the habit of having a video catch up over Facebook Messenger once a month or so. The next time we spoke, he informed me that Jane had read the sonnet beautifully at his wedding. Several people reported getting something in their eyes, making them water, as she did so.

I suppose that was appropriate.

Vile Jelly

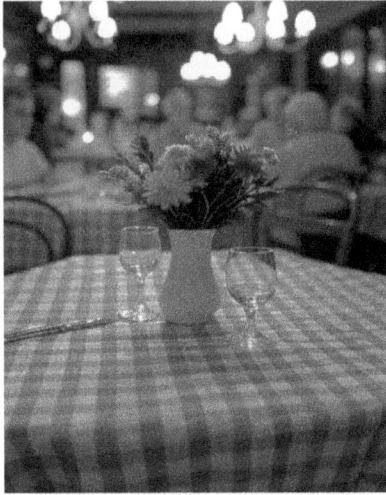

Chapter 10—The Ice Pack Cometh

'YOU WORRY TOO much, lah,' my doctor said, half smiling.

She had just taken my pressures. They were fine, although they were slightly higher than ideal. We had been chatting at the end of my appointment and I had mentioned that I dreaded these occasions, that they caused me endless anxiety in the day or two leading up to them. It had always been the case. Back home, every time a letter arrived telling me that I had to go the clinic on such-and-such a day at such-and-such a time, I felt my gut tighten. The interval between that moment and the appointment itself was one of trying to put it to the back of my mind. I was not too successful. The appointment was always there, like a little imp following me around, destroying my peace. I was not sure what I was so bothered about; the appointment would be what it would be.

My appointments from Taipan came through by text and were much more frequent than they had been back home—every six weeks to three months—but the effect was the same.

'You have a cataract forming in your right eye,' the doctor added nonchalantly.

'What?' I half-gasped, 'Aren't you supposed to be old to get those?'

'You can get them at any age,' she said.

'Oh my God!' I mock-moaned, 'My eyes are so rubbish! Can you replace them with someone else's please?'

'It is very slight at the moment,' she reassured me, 'As I say. You worry too much.'

Perhaps. Perhaps not. To be honest, I was not really sure where everything stood at that point. I had not had a fields test in Malaysia and it was now getting on for a year since my last one. I had not had a scan either. Moreover, my left eye was still a problem. Its pressure refused to equalize with that in my right eye.

On my next visit, it was discovered that it had pushed through the twenty mark.

'I'm going to try some different eye drops,' the doctor said.

'Okay,' I replied.

'I'm going to put you on Azopt and Tapcom. The Tapcom is preservative free and will need to be refrigerated.'

'Oh, right.'

'Your eyes are still very dry.'

'Like my sense of humour,' I said, feebly.

She looked at me as at a fool. I unwisely doubled down.

'I've always been a dry 'un. Actually, I've always been Adrian, but what's a vowel shift between friends?'

There was a pause.

'As I was saying,' she went on coolly, 'Your eyes are dry, so I am going to prescribe some medicinal gel. Put it in before you go to sleep. It will help to keep your eyes moist.'

So now I had to take three drops. I went to pick up my prescription note from the front desk.

'That will be three hundred ringgits please,' the young woman sitting there told me.

'No. No,' I said, 'I'm covered—I get insurance through my employer.'

'Yes,' she said, patiently, 'But the insurance only pay up to five hundred ringgits. Everything beyond that, you have to cover.'

More than a little unhappy, I reached for my Malaysian debit card, which, for some reason, was emblazoned with the crest of Barcelona Football Club. I wondered why the same consultation that I had been having for months suddenly cost me more. Presumably, the price included that of the medicines. They were not completely free to me after all! When I was eventually given fields tests and scans, my contribution would go up to at least eight hundred ringgits a visit. No wonder the tests were only offered occasionally!

I took the note to the pharmacy and repaired to Starbucks while waiting for the GL. When I returned, I was surprised to be given a bag containing the drops and an ice pack. The Tapcom did not come in a bottle, but a box. Each dose had its own little plastic ampule. There were thirty in a box. Thirty ampules for thirty days. The ice pack was placed alongside the box. I had not expected the requirement for refrigeration to be quite so big a deal.

'How long will the ice pack last?' I asked the young man behind the counter.

'About three hours,' he informed me.

'Can I go for lunch?' I asked.

'Yes,' he said, 'as long as you get the Tapcom into a fridge within about three hours.'

I took a Grab to KLCC and headed up to the main food court, which was called Signatures. I sat at the bar of a sushi restaurant. The bag filled with eye drops and ice was an encumbrance, but I stowed it at my feet the better to keep the counter in front of me free. The multi-coloured dishes of fish, rice and edamame beans passed before me on a conveyor belt, going round and round. A good metaphor for glaucoma, I thought.

The next time I went to Taipan, it was to learn that my left eye was still being troublesome. So I was placed on a regime of taking the Azopt three times a day and the Tapcom once in the evening. I could not help thinking that it would not be the last adjustment to my medication.

I fell into a new pattern based around a steady accumulation of polythene ice packs. My visits to Taipan were more frequent than my appointments because I had to pick up a prescription every thirty days regardless of whether the doctor had checked me out or not. I tended to go to the pharmacy on Saturdays, followed by lunch at one of the city centre's malls, usually Suria KLCC or Pavilion, Bukit Bintang. The latter had the advantage of being right next to an MRT station that was my pipeline back to Kajang. There was a strict time limit to how long I could remain in KL: the melting ice was insistent. The Tapcom had to be in my room and in my fridge within three hours, or my eyes would turn to pumpkins or something.

This was all manageable—until I needed to travel abroad, as was demanded by both my job and my desire to take advantage of living in South East Asia by, as it were, seeing a few of the sights. For example, when I took a trip to Bangkok to meet up with my friend Russ and his family (they had travelled from Dubai where they were living), the flight lasted for two hours. But that was extended by the need to arrive at the airport an appropriate interval before boarding and then to spend more time getting through immigration at the other end. That is before even considering the game of 'why doesn't my bag ever come out first' that I had no choice but to play at the baggage reclaim carousel. The Tapcom stood to be outside of a refrigerator for much of a day—long enough to render it useless. In planning the trip, I expended much energy on trying to find a way around this potentially disastrous issue.

In the end, I bought a thermos flask from Tesco, had it filled with ice at the hall of residence's bar the night before I set off and stored it in my fridge before adding the number of ampules that I would require the morning of departure. The flask could then simply be packed with my check-in luggage and retrieved when I reached my destination. This worked well enough for short flights. But longer journeys were more of a challenge.

In the summer of 2019, I planned to return to the UK for a couple of weeks. With a connection in Dubai, I would be travelling for around twenty-four hours when the pre- and post-travel periods were factored in. I searched everywhere for a flask that would guarantee to keep its contents cold for that long, but I could find nothing. Clearly, at the very least, I would have to carry the flask on to the plane. The trick would be to keep it as cold as possible for as long as possible so that the ice inside would not melt and leave me with a few bits of plastic floating around in lukewarm water as their precious contents were rendered ineffective.

Having checked in, I took the flask into one of the airport's toilets. Opening it and upending it over a sink released an alarming amount of water. A lot of the ice had already gone and I was only a couple of hours into the journey. Fortunately, this was not difficult to remedy. I went into a café and asked a barista whether he would mind giving me a top-up. He didn't and the status quo ante was restored. That bought more time. But the moment when I would need to board was coming up. I calculated that I could do another top-up in Dubai. The drops would be fine until then. Of course, I would have to explain what the flask was for as I took it through Security...

Surprisingly, this was not a problem. Neither was taking the flask on board the plane. Everyone I encountered was understanding and amenable to whatever requests I made. Sitting in my seat, I reflected on how easy it had been to solve the refrigeration problem, although that did not reduce the irritation that I felt at having to solve it in the first place.

When Karen met me at Birmingham Airport, I scrounged one last scoop of ice at a branch of a major café chain before we left.

Another way in which the Tapcom constrained me was around the timing of drop applications. I was restricted to home, or near to home, until after I had put the stuff in. This was not as simple as saying, well, just take it early if you have to. My doctor in Malaysia had advised me that the eyes are more receptive at specific times of day, 9pm being optimum. This was not very helpful. Not many films, for example, start that late and events such as concerts, gigs and parties would be out of the question. I defied my doctor's advice by taking the evening doses between six thirty and seven, but even that was a nuisance. I needed to be close to my fridge at that hour every night.

During my trip back to the UK, Karen and I drove to Staffordshire to see my Mum and her husband and we all decided to go out into the countryside to visit the National Memorial Arboretum. This was a park at which statues commemorating the actions of Britain's armed forces were arranged around extensive landscaped grounds. The monuments varied between the huge and the more human in scale. It was a place in which being alone with one's thoughts was the main activity. It was, furthermore, another primarily visual experience. Wandering around looking at ingenious installations themed around different regiments, medical support units and those who had been shot at dawn during the First World War, I was reminded again that my own capacity to participate even in something as undemanding as this was likely to diminish.

The night before my flight back to Malaysia, Karen and I met Tosh and Sharon for dinner. We rendezvoused at a French restaurant in the centre of Nottingham. Karen and I drove, Tosh and Sharon took a bus. Tosh was Sharon's de facto carer. She gripped his arm as he guided her, offering a running commentary of potential hazards. They had left the guide dog at home.

Inside, the restaurant had an authentic French feel, being small, welcoming and unpretentious. The table was covered with a checked tablecloth. Smooth jazz played through the sound system. The waitress was herself French. She gave us *les cartes* and took our orders. In line with the old-fashioned charm of the place, she used a note pad, not an iPad, to record what we wanted: steaks cooked 'blue' for Tosh and me, something vegetarian for Karen and a chicken dish for Sharon. We had a carafe of white wine.

As I poured us all a glass, I asked Tosh how he and Sharon were getting on.

'Fine,' he answered, 'the dog's all right.'

'Yes,' I said, 'I notice that she isn't with you.'

'Too much trouble, mate,' he said. 'You usually have to have an argument about it.'

I sipped my wine.

'I would have thought that they would be okay about it here,' I said.

'We can't take the risk,' Sharon said.

The conversation moved on. I asked Tosh what he was doing for a job since leaving the school.

'I've got some private tuition,' he told me, 'and I'm working for a company that provides language training online.'

'That's perfect for you,' Karen said, 'What about Sharon?'

'I was working for a charity dedicated to blindness,' she said, 'doing secretarial work.'

'She's a fucking amazing typist!' Tosh said, 'But the charity apparently likes doing everything for blind people apart from employ them.'

'Oh,' I said, 'Why is that?'

'They got rid of her and appointed a sighted person instead.'

'That's unfair,' Karen said.

'Too right!' Tosh agreed.

'Did you do anything wrong?' I asked Sharon tentatively.

'No,' she said, 'They just didn't renew my contract.'

Both Tosh and Sharon qualified for disability allowances from the government, but that amounted to not much more than a safety net—it did not guarantee a high quality of life. Some other form of income was required. The conversation confirmed the difficulty of procuring that if you are visually impaired. I could understand why Tosh deferred back to the Equalities Act so often!

As the meal drew to an end, we asked the waitress to take the obligatory Facebook picture. I looked on my phone at what came back. I was gazing enthusiastically at the lens, Karen looked distracted, Tosh was staring vaguely in my direction and Sharon seemed to not be aware that a picture was being taken.

If anyone had wanted to measure how much vision everyone present enjoyed, that photograph would have been all that they would have needed.

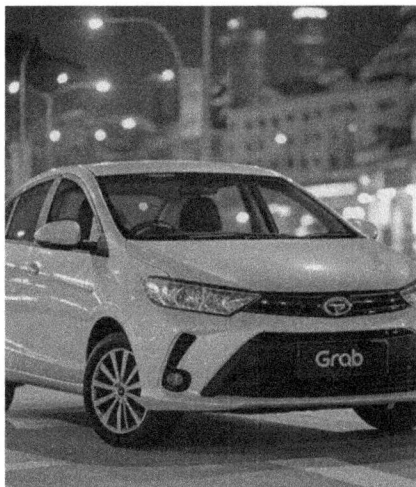

Chapter 11—The Moonlight Pharmacy

THAT CHRISTMAS, KAREN came out to visit me and we spent the week at Traders Hotel in KL. A place that enjoyed some fame by dint of its 'sky bar' having been rated the best in South East Asia, it allowed us to live in style as we took advantage of everything the city had to offer. I was waiting to check in to our room when Karen – who was on her way out at the time - called me from Dubai. I took that as emblematic of how far my life had changed in the recent past. To be waiting in a queue at a top hotel in Malaysia talking to my wife who was in the Middle East was something that I could scarcely have imagined even a couple of years earlier. Yet there we were.

However, things were not quite as perfect as that picture makes them seem. Karen's mother had recently passed away. Outwardly, Karen was handling this with characteristic fortitude, but I was concerned about her mental health. Over the course of her stay, it became clear that she was suffering more than she was letting on. We spent New Year's Eve in the coastal kampung of Bagan Lalang, which, some unbelievably good seafood restaurants aside, is not a lively part of the world. Even those restaurants were not much use to vegetarian

Karen. It was hardly a recipe for cheering her up.

Dropping her off at the airport a day or two later, I resolved to make more of a success of her next visit.

That visit never happened.

In early 2020 news began to filter out of China of a new coronavirus that was affecting the province of Wuhan. Before long it acquired the name COVID-19. It appeared to have fatal consequences for a large percentage of those who contracted it.

Initially, I saw no reason to regard it as much of a threat. Yes, Malaysia was not a million miles from China, but this was not the first time that such a thing had happened. On previous occasions, diseases had considerately remained firmly within the borders of their country of origin. I saw COVID-19 as someone else's problem.

Then it was reported in Singapore. That was closer. Worryingly closer. I was due to travel down there to do some teaching. There was a debate in the office about whether I should go. In the end, I did, but, while I was there, it emerged that someone who worked in the same building in which I was based had caught the disease. On my return to Malaysia, I was told to stay away from the office and work from the hall of residence for two weeks.

It is a measure of the growing air of paranoia that I was even vaguely regarded as being at risk. Firstly, when I say 'building in which I was based' I mean 'gigantic complex through which several thousand people passed daily'. Secondly, my lessons took place at the weekends, when the infected person would have been somewhere else. But all kinds of rumours were swirling around about how the virus could be transmitted. You didn't need to be close to a sufferer it was said—the virus remained on objects, such as doorknobs, for an indeterminate period. What if I had inadvertently spent time in a room that had been entered by the infected person? Or pressed a lift button that he or she had used? I would be as good as dead.

In all honesty, the two weeks of my quarantine were good fun. The cafes, restaurants and snack bars in the hall of residence were all open to me and setting myself up in the 'study area' with my iPad was an agreeable change to sitting at my desk in the office all day. On one occasion, my colleague and friend PK came over for lunch. On another, two female colleagues, Sharlin and Suria, bought me some deluxe cookies (complete with teddy bear!) as a way to show me that they were thinking of me.

Things were not to be that good again.

COVID-19 continued to spread. The number of cases rose by the day. Some countries were hit worse than others, but almost all were affected to some extent. Panicked governments looked for ways to contain the disease. People were dying! By the thousand! Europe effectively closed down. First Italy, then Denmark, declared themselves quarantined on a national scale. Others soon followed. All across the continent, public gatherings—at which the risk of infection was highest—were banned or voluntarily suspended. Film premieres—including that for the new James Bond outing—were postponed. Sporting programmes—La Liga, the Premier League, F1, the Cheltenham Festival—were massively disrupted. To my chagrin, the release of Deep Purple's new album was pushed back by two months.

Travel was restricted—there would be no more trips to Singapore for a while, or, indeed, anywhere else. The USA placed a moratorium on flights from Europe, as it, too, drew up measures to restrict people's movements. The World Health Organisation declared a pandemic. A new phrase, 'social distancing' entered the lexicon. This referred to remaining as far as possible from other human beings, which was, it was believed, the best way to avoid infection. It led to the emergence of some bizarre practices, such as the replacement of the handshake with a less intimate bump of the elbows.

Before long, people were forbidden to leave their homes at all, except in an emergency. To be sure, not everyone was unhappy with the situation. Tosh's response was, 'Social distancing? What's not to like?' My sister declared it 'a life goal realised.'

The so-called 'Great Lockdown' began sometime around April 2020. The entire world closed for business. Cinemas, bars, clubs—all pulled down their shutters. Pictures of deserted city centres—Rome! Venice! Madrid!—started to appear on social media.

All but essential shops (supermarkets, banks and—thank God—

pharmacies) were ordered not to open. Airports became ghost towns. Roads emptied of traffic. Office blocks were mothballed. Grass began to grow on abandoned streets.

Those who could work from home were told to do so. This included me and I began a miserable few months of sitting in my room with only my iPad for company. Those who could not work from home were forced to wait it out, knowing that every day that they spent doing nothing was a day closer to their jobs vanishing altogether. Shopping became a surreal experience.

Malaysia took a particularly stern line. Not only was everything put into suspended animation, but travel was only permitted if absolutely necessary and only then up to a radius of ten kilometres from home. For longer journeys, should they be unavoidable, written permission had to obtained from the police—or, at least, some sort of explanatory documentation had to be provided. The name given to lockdown was officially MCO, or Movement Control Order.

Signing in was required to enter any public space. The idea, I suppose, was to allow you to be contacted if someone else in there at around the same time was found to be positive for the virus. This never happened to me, even when the more high-tech version—the MySejahtera smartphone app—came online. This generated a QR code that could be scanned by the ever-present COVID gatekeepers at any location. It also kept a running total of cases in the country on any given day.

As for reaching Taipan: it was a good deal further than ten kilometres away from where I was living. That was, in itself, a problem, but, since the hospital was now the frontline of the COVID war, the chances of my appointments being anyone's highest priority were low.

A cameo of the new reality would be the day on which I was forced to top up my reserves of cash and headed to Tesco. On reaching the shop, I was confronted with a socially distanced queue of people that snaked away from the main door and into the car park; a strict limit had been placed on the number of customers allowed in at any one moment. After fifty restless minutes, I reached the front and entered, having signed in and had my temperature taken by having a Star Trek phaserlike device pointed at my forehead (this was to become a constant of the period, too). The outlets that clustered around the main shop like benign parasites were closed. Fortunately, the bank ATMs were working. In Tesco itself, everything seemed weirdly normal. Nothing had been sold out, apart from anti-bacterial wipes, which everywhere had become as rare as living dinosaurs.

I consoled myself by thinking that the hall of residence would not be such a bad place to pass lockdown. The cafes, the snack bars, the shop—they would make the experience much more bearable. No such luck. Gripped by a zeal that made the rest of the country seem lax by comparison, the management removed every element that could even vaguely encourage social contact. Chairs were taken away and stacked in a blocked-off corner, tables were piled one on top of the other. The gym—which was not a free perk—was locked up. Even the benches in the garden disappeared. The back gate that had served as the quickest route by which to access campus was padlocked. The only way in and out was through the main entrance, which meant gaining clearance from the ever-present security guards. It was still possible to buy hot food, but it was served in take away tubs for consumption in individual rooms. With some horror, I realised that I was, to all intents and purposes, in prison. Most of the students, sensing that this was coming, had headed back home in the brief interval before the most draconian rules were put in place. The compound was all but empty. A few people stayed, but they were little in evidence.

The big challenge, of course, was how to ensure a steady supply of eye drops. Almost as soon as the lockdown was declared, I received a text from Taipan cancelling an appointment that was looming. I was kind of expecting that, but there was no indication of for when it would be rescheduled.

I had a small stock of the drops, so, in the immediate term, there was no need to panic. But the chief virtue of the Tapcom was that it gave me a precise measure of how long I had. Around forty days. If the lockdown lasted more than a month or so, I would be in a potentially disastrous position. Added jeopardy came from the difficulty I had with sourcing the drops from elsewhere. Phone calls to two or three of the pharmacies in the vicinity confirmed that, while Azopt was readily available, Tapcom was not. I would have little choice but to procure it, at least in the short term, from Taipan.

As the amounts of each medicine diminished, I felt myself become more and more tense. I was hearing stories of people being turned back on roads as they tested the ten kilometre limit. The police (often backed up with rifle-toting soldiers) were prone to carrying out spot checks that were causing long traffic tailbacks in the city. Even if I could prove that I was doing something legitimate, there was no guarantee that I would be given passage.

Eventually, the day came on which there was no further putting the matter off. I contacted Taipan and asked if they could send me a doctor's note. They obliged and a scan of a handwritten prescription arrived as an email attachment. For added authority, I asked the University doctor to do likewise; she was equally helpful. With two supporting documents saved to my phone, I felt confident that I could get through, but I really had no idea what to expect. I had been stuck in the hall of residence for weeks by this stage. My hair—such as it was—had grown out of control and my beard was beginning to make me look like Gandalf the Wizard.

So, one midweek morning I found myself by the compound's main entrance bleakly summoning a Grab. To my amazement, the app came back straight away to let me know that a suitable ride was already there. It was a car parked directly across the road from where I was standing. The driver got out.

'You want to go to Taipan?' he asked.

'Yes,' I confirmed.

'Do you have a permission letter?'

I showed him the two doctors' notes. He seemed satisfied. But I had an altogether different worry. What if I got there, was dropped off and got my medicines, only to find that no cab driver was willing to come all the way out to the hall of residence to deliver me back home? The MRT was not an option—that was not running.

'Listen,' I said to the driver, 'Would you be willing to wait at the other end to bring me back?'

He said that he was happy to do so, but I felt that more information was only fair.

'But you might have to hang around for as long as an hour,' I told him, anticipating the wait for the GL.

'That's okay, boss' he said.

Business must have been slow—hence his sitting in his car outside the hall in the hope of a student coming out looking for a lift to somewhere or other. I climbed nervously into the back seat and clicked the seat belt clasp into place. The car set off.

There was none of the banter that was the norm for Grab rides. I was not asked where I was from or what Premier League team I support (for the record, I support Birmingham City, who are not in the Premier League). Both myself and the driver had over us the lugubrious lustre of people living through war time. Pulling out on to the road into the city revealed a predictably quiet landscape. But not one that was completely devoid of life. Other cars were making journeys. Not many, for sure, but more than I would have expected. The traffic lights worked as they always did. It all felt strangely—well—unstrange. All rather normal, in fact. We passed through the straggling buildings at the edge of town without encountering anything out of the ordinary. As we reached the main highway, I was thinking that it could have been any average day.

I was conscious, though, that we were heading over the notional ten-kilometre line. Were we to be stopped from now on, I would have some fast talking to do. I feared a roadblock at any second. None appeared.

We entered the outskirts of the city. Still nothing. All the stories that I had been told about what was going on were proving to be spectacularly off the mark. As the car turned into the hilly road leading up to the hospital's main entrance, I was almost complacent. Almost. A big part of me wondered how long my luck would hold.

'Are you happy to wait?' I asked again.

The driver gave me a thumbs up. He handed me a piece of paper on which he had scribbled his mobile number.

'Okay. I will give you a call when I am ready to leave,' I said, 'As I say, it might be as long as an hour.'

'No problem, boss,' he replied.

Most of the doors to the hospital were locked. There was only one way in and to get through that I had to have my temperature taken by a device on a tripod. The masked nurses—looking like figures from a dystopian sci-fi film—got the reading they were looking for and I was ushered in.

It was not the Taipan to which I had become accustomed. The shops and food stalls were closed. No Starbucks today! The lounge area was an open expanse with not a chair in sight. I walked around to the pharmacy and showed the prescription on my phone. I had a decision to make. I could wait for the GL—which would be a pretty grim thing to do in the hospital as it was. Or I could just pay for the medicines out of my own pocket and get moving. The latter would not exactly be cheap, but it would be quick. Since I could not firmly rely on my Grab driver to honour his commitment, I opted to pay.

With a bag of eye drops and an ice pack gripped firmly in my hand, I called the driver. He was waiting outside the main entrance. I climbed into the car. There was no need for words. We both felt like we were about to run the gauntlet of some ill-defined, but implacable, enemy. We headed out towards the highway. It was quiet. The opposite carriageway, the one that led into the city, was clogged with a long line of traffic caused by police performing spot checks. Had I set off only half an hour later, I would have been stuck in that. I somehow began to feel that I was being smiled upon by a higher power.

We were soon enough back in the countryside. Then Kajang. Then the hall of residence. Home! Without once running into a problem. The whole expedition had taken an unlikely two hours. Neither doctor's note had been required. I paid the Grab driver and headed into my room, grateful that I had avoided the worst.

But: that could not be the way to do this every time. Acquiring my eye drops may have been easier than expected, but the second I put the box of Tapcom in my fridge, the clock was ticking again. My only option was to try a pharmacy within the ten-kilometre zone. Most had already disappointed, but there was one that I had not really explored: Moonlight Pharmacy. It was located in the centre of the local town, so was no more than a few minutes drive away by Grab. I had, in fact, called it already, but the person who answered had not, apparently, understood what I was saying and the conversation ended on a rather inconclusive note. I tried again. This time, the news was good. Yes, they could supply both Azopt and Tapcom. No, I would not need a new prescription.

Perfect!

As my drops began to run out, I ordered some replacements and went to collect them in the obligatory Grab. I discovered that the pharmacy was in a row of shops—built in the utilitarian concrete style that was the vernacular around there—that in normal times, would have been bustling. The parking area in front of them would have been packed. Not so now. The pharmacy, being essential, was the only shop trading. The car park was empty. The road deserted. It was all disconcertingly reminiscent of the opening scene of *28 Days Later*.

Inside, the pharmacy was basic in design, but well-stocked. The main counter was a barrier to a door out to the back in which most of the prescription medicines were kept. I gave my details to the young woman waiting patiently behind the counter. She put me in mind of a character from a Beckett play. She disappeared through the door and returned a minute or two later with both sets of drops. The Tapcom was not paired with an ice pack.

'Has that been stored in a fridge?' I asked, pointing to it.

The young woman vaguely nodded 'yes'. I was not so sure, but what could I do? I had to take it as it was. A bonus was a little basket containing bottles of antibacterial handwash on the counter. These were still nigh on unobtainable anywhere else, yet they were freely available here at a very reasonable price. I bought a couple.

If my tribulations were bad, however, they were as nothing compared to Tosh's. He developed a detached retina. This happens when the thin layer of light sensitive material at the back of the eye peels away from its supporting wall. Symptoms include the thread-like chimeras known as floaters and dark curtains passing across the vision. If a corrective operation is not carried out urgently, blindness can be the result.

It first manifested itself for Tosh when he was reading a book called

Vile Jelly

Mentality Monsters: How Jurgen Klopp Took Liverpool FC From Also-Rans to Champions of Europe by Paul Tomkins. He began to notice the telltale signs in his left eye. He made it to the end of Mr Tomkins' musings, but, as he somewhat ruefully explained, it was the last hard copy book that he ever read and there will be no others.

His doctor made no bones about the seriousness of the situation: 'Do nothing,' he said, 'and you go blind in your left eye—and since you don't exactly have a great deal of sight to start with, we can't let that happen.'

Tosh had surgery as soon as possible, silicon oil being used to repair the breaks. Nurses were on strike that day, so only emergency cases were being admitted—but Tosh was an emergency case. Following the operation, he had to 'posture' for ten days by lying as still as possible in bed. For ten days. Small breaks were allowed. These amounted to a few minutes in any given hour. It was a personal lockdown for him. But, as Liverpool had just won their first football championship since Adam was a lad, Tosh was generally quite cheerful.

In Malaysia we lapsed into a pattern of hope being quickly dashed by despair. As the number of daily cases on MySejahtera declined, the longed-for easing of restrictions became more probable. It never happened completely. The Great Lockdown ended with shops and restaurants reopening—sort of. The numbers who were permitted to enter any given public area were limited, so waiting in a queue was the default for anyone wishing to get out of their house.

Travel bans were still in place. The Malaysian government had placed the UK on a list of countries from which incoming passengers were not permitted, so Karen was unable to visit me. I could have visited her, but were I to have done so, I might not have been able to come back. We were stuck on opposite sides of the world, with only Facebook Messenger to connect us. Months stretched to a year, then to nearly a year and a half. We were never physically in each other's presence during that time.

Worse, the cases reported on MySejahtera, having bottomed out, began to rise again. It was not a constant rate. Some days, the headline number dropped a little, but the trend was upwards and, as these things are wont to do, it accelerated. Before too long, the threshold for another lockdown was reached.

I was back to staying in my room and acquiring my medicines from Moonlight Pharmacy. That would not have been too much of a hardship, but my contract was reaching its end and, for all sorts of reasons, not least the separation from Karen, I was not inclined to renew it. The lockdown eased and it seemed like a good time to head home.

The luck that I had enjoyed on previous occasions did not hold. As I began to make my preparations to leave Malaysia, MySejahtera's remorseless logic kicked in yet again. A lockdown every bit as severe as those that we had been enduring for so long was coming back and I was due to fly home right in the middle of it.

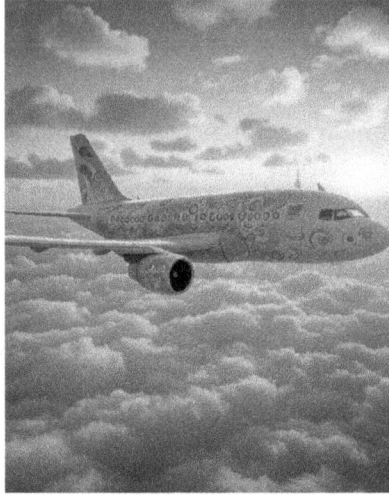

Chapter 12—Back Home

'WHY DO YOU want to come back into a secondary school having worked in a university?'

The speaker was the Director of Studies at a school in Dubai with which I was trying to get a job. We were speaking over Microsoft Teams. It was in my room in Malaysia. It was a couple of months before my contract was due to expire.

'I suppose it comes down to the difference between your job and your profession,' I said, 'My job is working in Educational Leadership—and it's great—but my passion, my profession, is English language and literature. That's the thing I have devoted myself to.'

This answer impressed him.

'That's what we are looking for—people who are passionate about their subjects.'

'That's me,' I confirmed.

After that initial conversation, I went through the usual application process and received an offer. I was given twenty-four hours to accept. In a piece of unplanned synchronicity with Malaysia, the school was a remote outpost of a prominent institution in England. Beyond that, the similarities between the two were minimal.

In many ways, my good fortune in landing the job was not without its disadvantages. These mainly revolved around the types of preparation that were necessary for me to take up the offer. For example, the Dubai government required me to get certificates of good conduct from every country in which I had lived. The list consisting of precisely two was lucky, but in order to obtain one from Malaysia, I had to go to the administrative capital of Putrajaya, which was—obviously—more than ten kilometers away from my room.

Booking my flight was also not the straightforward operation it should have been. I knew that, on my arrival back in the UK, I would have to quarantine for ten days. In the best-case scenario, that would be in my own home at no cost. But, if I landed in a 'red list' country en route, I would have to hole up in a government-approved hotel for a fee of seventeen hundred pounds.

'Red list' countries were those that the British government had decided, for no clear reason, were so decimated by COVID that merely setting foot inside them was to risk infection. Even connecting at an airport was regarded as sufficient to merit the hotel sanction. Malaysia was okay—it was only 'amber list'—but pretty much every country between it and the UK was red. Thus, I was unable to take any airline that connected in the UAE, Qatar, Oman, India... Singapore was amber list, but so what? Flying there would probably only be the first of two connections, the second of which would almost certainly have the near two-grand price tag attached.

I scanned available flights with an ever-greater sense of despair, until...I found one that would work for me. KLM, the Dutch carrier, had a route that went from KL to Singapore to Amsterdam to Birmingham with ne'er a stop in a red list country. It was ideal, except...the necessity for eye drop refrigeration. Singapore to Amsterdam was a twelve-hour leg. Add to that a rapid turnaround in Amsterdam and the Tapcom could well be in an unrefrigerated state for a good portion of the journey.

Before I got to that, I paid my final visit to Taipan. It was about a week before I was due to fly. I had a scan and a fields test. The doctor told me that the latter revealed the vision in my left eye to be 'about 50%', while my right eye was 'at least 80%'. Low pressures were also a big plus. The scan was glossed over somewhat. Still, the future was bright—to use yet another image of sight. I had glaucoma, yes, but it could have been worse. The major symptom was under control and there was every reason to assume that I could get on with my life unhindered. Tosh made the good point that perception is important in these matters. As he said, he, on his best day, had never come close to 50% in either eye, never mind eighty. In his own colourful words, 'If I woke up tomorrow morning with 50% on my left eye, I'd feel like Steve Austin.'

Nonetheless, as I left her office, the doctor warned me.

'You are heading towards an operation.'

I was unprepared for this, but I assumed that she did not mean imminently. I mentally pictured a drawn and wasted future me being wheeled into an operating theatre, ready to have blades and needles applied to the most delicate parts of my face.

As far as leaving Malaysia was concerned, I could do nothing without a COVID test. In order to legally enter the UK, I had to fill in a 'passenger locator form'—to confirm who I was and where I would be staying—which was easy enough. But I had to test negative not more than three days (or 72 hours—I was never really sure which) before I flew. The tests could be carried out by the University's doctor and the results would be available twenty-four hours later—in theory.

I was booked on to a Friday night flight. No problem, then: I could get the test on Wednesday and receive the results on Thursday. Even if they were a bit late, they should still have arrived in plenty of time. Except that I couldn't do that, because Malaysia was having one of its frequent public holidays on the Wednesday; no tests were going to be carried out that day. Consulting the relevant (British) YouGov website, I discovered that it was possible to get a test on Tuesday if I were flying on Friday, but my test would be on Tuesday morning, while my flight did not take off until 9pm on Friday—which would break the 72-hour rule (if there were a 72 hour rule and I thought it best to assume that there was...). If I waited until Thursday to have the test, the result might not be available before I needed to leave for the airport.

What to do? In the end, I decided to have tests on both Tuesday and Thursday, each being the other's failsafe, so to speak. It was an expensive course of action and one which resulted in more than a few raised eyebrows among the staff at the University's clinic, but what else could I do?

The swab that the University doctor shoved up my nose went all the way in: I did not know that my nose cavity extended that far back. I am not entirely convinced that she did not get a bit of brain tissue. To call it painful would be an understatement.

Then there was the Tapcom dilemma. I had experimented with putting the flask filled with ice in my fridge. It served to extend the life of the ice. That was my only option: take the flask on board with me and hope that the stewardesses would be prepared to store it in the same place as the Business Class white wine.

On the day, I was dropped off at the airport by a couple of colleagues. A MCO was in full force, so our plans to have lunch were more or less stymied. We had a rather glum pizza in the hall of residence's outdoor barbecue area, which had somehow survived the chair purge. Four of us sat around a table eating our last meal together. On the way, we stopped at a mall just outside the airport's perimeter. I have rarely felt so depressed to be in such a place. There were so few customers that I was not sure it was even open when we pulled into the car park. Signing in was mandatory, of course, as was having our body temperatures taken. Inside, most shops were closed. The only way to get a drink or something to eat was on a 'take away' basis: we were forced to stand around in the passageways with our coffees.

Only passengers were admitted to the airport, so I said goodbye to my colleagues of four years by the main door. The airport was quiet, nearly deserted. Some hardy cafes and restaurants were soldiering gamely on, but, as in the mall, their products could only be consumed in public areas. I ended up spending a couple of hours leaning against a wall longing for boarding to start.

Eventually, it did and I ambled along the connecting bridge to the plane. Other passengers were in short supply. At least I had most of

Economy to myself. The change in Singapore was only to re-equip and re-fuel, so I would be staying on board all the way to Amsterdam. I asked a stewardess if she could put my flask in a fridge. Pleasingly, the answer was 'yes', although it did not go into a fridge so much as a 'cool cabinet'. It was better than nothing.

Singapore was only forty-five minutes away, so I, along with my fellow travellers, were corralled into a small part of one of Changi Airport's terminals during the brief stop off. There are not many places on earth in which I would rather connect in most circumstances. That day, it was another exercise in mental endurance. The terminal's interior was so lifeless that it may well have developed an echo.

Back on the plane, there were more passengers. The in-flight entertainment was inaccessible because, naturally, headphones fell foul of lockdown restrictions. I looked forward glumly to a dull journey. It proved not to be so. The flight was remarkably smooth. I had a row to myself and I relaxed with the supplied blanket and pillow. I felt at peace. I reflected on my time in Malaysia. It had been an adventure, an adventure that was coming to an end. Still, there was another just around the corner. Being alone with your thoughts is fine when your thoughts are good ones.

Schiphol Airport in Amsterdam was relatively lively, albeit that it was not at its busiest. Birmingham was another soul-destroying void, but Karen met me there and we headed back to Nottingham for the beginning of my quarantine period.

It was good to see her. Our separation had been for far too long. Our life together could finally begin for real. In the UK, some restrictions were still in place, but the country was rousing itself from the pandemic slumber. I just had to get through the ten days of something like house arrest that stretched before me. Taking self-administered COVID tests was obligatory. I did not stick the swab as far up my nose as the University doctor had done.

It was the end of May. Karen and I were scheduled to fly out to Dubai in the middle of August. I could see little point in trying to get a glaucoma appointment during what was, effectively, an extended layover. The Tapcom in the flask would last until well into July and I also had a sound stock of Azopt. That gave me plenty of time in which to source an interim supply.

Among my first calls in the UK was Tosh. Once my quarantine was over, we met for lunch in the centre of Nottingham. This was the occasion on which a small tradition started—of having a couple of beers (mine a boring lager, Tosh's a real ale called The Horse's Cock, or something similar), followed by a large fish, chip, mushy pea and battered sausage lunch at a place called Moulin Rouge.

It was a mild June day, so we ended up sitting at a table outside a branch of a well-known café chain. Much of our conversation was around England's remarkable performance in the Euro 2020 football competition, which, as its name suggests, happened in 2021. We turned to more personal matters. I sipped my Americano as Tosh said:

'The operation has been a success, mate.'

'Good,' I replied.

'Yeah—posturing was a bit fucking boring, but at least it meant that I could listen to a lot of music.'

'That was with Alexa?'

'Yeah.'

Alexa was the Amazon online music gateway. It was activated by saying, 'Alexa, play…' whatever. This did not quickly become grating. It did not quickly become grating at all.

'My quarantine was pretty tedious, too,' I said, 'Although I wrote a musical to keep me going.'

'Nice one!' Tosh said.

This was true. I had been commissioned to write the script and lyrics for a contemporary-set musical based on the Medieval morality play *Everyman*. I set it during the lockdown to give it added relevance.

'How's work?' I asked.

Tosh sipped his latte and puffed on his vape device.

'It's okay,' he said, 'I was away from it for a couple of weeks for posturing, but that's the great thing about being self-employed—or nearly self-employed—you can do that sort of thing without too much trouble.'

'Well, Karen and I will be heading off to Dubai soon,' I said.

'Looking forward to it?'

At that stage, I was a little uncertain. My job in Malaysia had brought me into contact with all manner of people and activities that went well beyond the basic remit of an academic. I had, for example, worked extensively with Academy of Sciences Malaysia, which, on one occasion, had called for me to attend a meeting at a hotel in Putrajaya at which top officials from every Malaysian ministry discussed a document of which I was co-author. At a conference in Yangon, Myanmar, I had sat on a panel with high-ranking members of the country's main education policy committee. To be heading back to a school to teach *An Inspector Calls* to fifteen-year-olds was an anti-climax, to say the least. But it was a good job and I was certainly excited at the prospect of life in Dubai.

'Mostly yes,' I said, 'I just hope that I can get the eye care that I need.'

'Shouldn't be a problem, mate,' Tosh said.

'I wouldn't have thought so,' I said, 'I get medical cover as part of my package.'

My preparations to leave were less fraught with uncertainty than had been the case with Malaysia. I had been hanging around for nearly four months before boarding my flight to KL, constantly doubting whether I would be going at all. Now, everything was well organised and I only had a few weeks between the end of my quarantine and departure for the Middle East. Much of this was spent doing the rounds of friends and family. I met up with some of my female ex-colleagues in Wisbech. I had lunch with my family on my sister's rather large country estate in Staffordshire. She showed us her ever-growing menagerie of hobby animals: pigs, sheep—a special breed of sheep—and ducks.

When the time came to replenish my eye drop supplies, I simply got a prescription from my doctor. I tried to get my prescriptions for free, my reason being that I was technically unemployed. Apparently, free prescriptions are only for certain types of unemployed people. Who knew? Some confusion was caused by the fact that Tapcom as such was not available. Something very similar was and I got that instead. It still needed to be refrigerated.

Karen was clearly ambivalent about the coming move. Our initial conversations about it had all happened during the dying days of my tenure in Malaysia and so had been at a distance. This had necessarily caused them to be less nuanced than they would have been had we been face-to-face. Because I received the offer while still in Malaysia, Karen had not been a significant part of the decision-making about whether to accept it—especially as I had only been given a twenty-four-hour window. She expressed her happiness to be going, but I could tell that she was nervous about what would be a huge change. Her university education aside, she had only previously lived in two places: her home city of Sheffield and her current place of abode, Nottingham. To be decamping quite so finally, not to mention suddenly, to somewhere thousands of miles away was a big step for her. I knew Dubai quite well, having visited on numerous occasions. I drew upon those experiences to reassure her that all would be well.

We travelled to Heathrow Airport the day before our flight and checked into an hotel. On the day, we stacked bags that had already been packed for some days by the front door and awaited the taxi. This was not the cheapest method of transport, but keeping things stress-free was important to us; in the event, the taxi was to provide a source of comically unexpected tension, but that was for our arrival at the airport.

Before that, we said goodbye to our neighbour Teresa, who had agreed to look after the house for us while we were away and to do things like check the post and so on. A complication was that one of the bedrooms was taken by a lodger, an associate professor at the University of Nottingham. He was something of a 'legacy' problem for me, as he had been around since before I moved in. He was Chinese and spent a good proportion of the year in his home country, while continuing to pay the rent. He thus represented a solid source of passive income. We could not in all conscience evict him. Teresa promised to ensure that he would not misuse the place, but it was with some misgivings that we left what was in every major respect our marital home in the sole possession of a near-stranger.

Karen and I sat in the back of the car as it took us down the motorway towards our meeting with destiny. We said little. At the airport, we were dropped off at our hotel and the taxi sped off. It turned out not to be our hotel, but a hotel with exactly the same name some miles from the one that we had booked. It took another taxi journey for us to reach the right hotel. I had the flask of eye drops topped up in the bar and stowed it in the fridge in our room.

That night, we had dinner in the restaurant. Over a glass of wine, we considered the escapade on which we were embarking. Karen's apprehensiveness was tempered by her much-attested resilience. I was still talking about my concerns over taking what I could only view as a professional step backwards. None of it boded all that well.

In a metaphorical sense, I had a clouded view of whatever we would find at the other end of our flight. More literally, I was becoming more and more aware of a blurring at the edges of the vision in my right eye.

It was not too serious as yet, but I could not forget the words of the doctor in Malaysia about the cataract that she had detected.

Sitting in that restaurant, looking out of the large windows towards the runways, I wondered whether I would even be able to read the books that I would be teaching to the pupils at my new school.

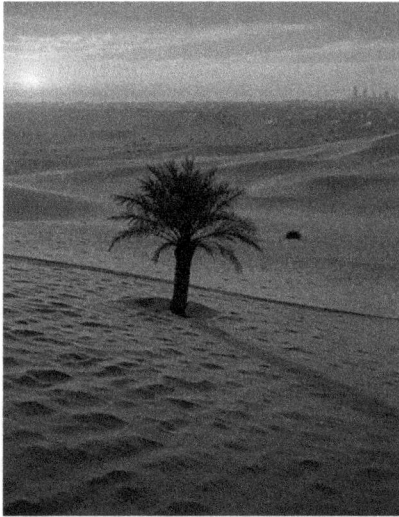

Chapter 13—The Lone and Level Sands

COVID RESTRICTIONS HAD by no means completely gone away and our time in Dubai was to be blighted by them.

The government of the UAE had a delicate balancing act to perform. They had spent a colossal amount of money preparing for the latest Expo, which they were hosting. Six-month long paeans to human progress, Expos were held every half decade, individual cities being their locations. They consisted of 'pavilions' supplied by participating nations. These varied in ambition. Those from smaller or poorer countries were not much more than museum exhibitions set up in standard spaces provided by the hosts. Others were bespoke architectural commissions that often resembled improbably luxurious university buildings (the one from Germany was actually called a 'campus'). National prestige was as much the motive as any desire to showcase global achievements.

Expo 2020, naturally enough for the 'new normal', took place between 2021 and 2022. Such a delay was bad enough. A new full lockdown would kill the event outright, causing a huge loss to the UAE both financially and reputationally. COVID infection rates, then, were played down and restrictions on personal movement were slight, even as other measures bordered on the draconian. Masks were mandatory and educational institutions were subject to constant no-notice visits from KHDA (the Knowledge and Human Development Agency) to ensure that all current rules were being complied with.

Karen and I were accommodated in an apartment a pleasant stroll from the racecourse and a short taxi ride from the main business area. Visually, we were met with the incredible every time we stepped outside. From the swimming pool of our block, the entire vista of Dubai city stretched out in front of us. During the day when it was partly obscured by heat and sand haze, it was only impressive, but at night... it became a futuristic fantasy of human potential. Luminescent skyscrapers jutted upwards from a polychromatic dreamscape. It was chutzpah embodied.

At the centre of it all stood the ultimate statement, the Burj Khalifa, the world's tallest building, pointing upwards like a needle that might puncture the moon. The towers that clustered around it like begging children would all, at a relatively recent date, have been unsurpassed for loftiness. Now, they looked small and slightly apologetic.

We quickly got into the habit of visiting the Dubai Mall, inside of which everything was designed for maximum visual impact. The main stores of the great fashion houses lined the walkways like Venetian palazzos, high, broad, sometimes quirky, almost always devoid of customers. The aquarium's main wall was a vast sheet of glass that gave a view of the manmade extract of blue ocean beyond with its plenitude of creatures in constant motion. The spine of a diplodocus skeleton curved upwards towards the ceiling of the area known as the Souk.

There was an attraction in the Mall called *Infinity Des Lumieres*. This was a cavernous hall that showed displays based on the work of artists— Van Gogh was in residence when we visited—using digital projections, animations and music. Apart from what this might say about gallery curation in the twenty first century, it was an experience that required good eyes. Karen and I walked around as projections of Van Gogh's self-portrait, or his chair, or his sunflowers, extracted from their contexts and superimposed on, say, one of his countryside paintings, drifted across a wall, while the floor beneath our feet transformed into a carpet of Impressionist flowers.

We spent the evenings in the cool of our apartment or at one of the cafes or restaurants nearby. We would often walk to the local branch of the supermarket Spinneys, which was so carefully stocked as to more resemble an art gallery in its own right than a food shop. Occasionally, we would go around to Russ's house for a drink or dinner. He lived with his family in a villa in a district called Arabian Ranches. Reaching it involved a taxi ride through a part of the desert, serene sands stretching far into the distance.

Finding an eye doctor was a priority. The small stock of drops that I had brought with me was running low. Most promising was a clinic on the edge of the Sheikh Zayed Road. The SZR, as it is often known, is in many ways Dubai's main artery. Indeed, it is the whole UAE's main artery, crossing the territory between the borders with Saudi Arabia at one of its ends and Oman at the other. It is very busy and, in the centre of the city, very wide, which made the rather modest set of clinics nestled next to it seem all the more ordinary. This was no Taipan. It was a functional and business-like facility. A place to be in and out of quickly.

The eye clinic was located on the first floor and consisted of a comfortable, if small, waiting area with consultation rooms leading from it. The reception desk was simple and, as was de rigeur in those days, protected by a transparent plastic screen. Upon registering for my first appointment, I was told to take a seat. Karen was with me.

We sat on a sofa with a panoramic view of the SZR. We were in one of those parts of Dubai where modern blocks mix with modest low-rise shops and cafes. Both feebly impose themselves on a desert that is the context to everything and which always gives the impression that it has only reluctantly yielded to these upstart humans and will eventually reclaim its rights with an overwhelming surge.

When I was called in, I was met with a doctor who was a stark contrast to the urbane woman from Malaysia. This guy wore his white coat like he had just picked it up from a charity shop. He was spectacularly bad tempered.

'Sit down,' he barked.

'How are you?' I asked in an ill-advised effort to bond.

'Mmm,' he mumbled gruffly.

I did as I was told and had my pressures taken. They were slightly up but were nothing to get too concerned about. The doctor, however, changed my drop prescription. This was because Tapcom was not available. He substituted it for something that—thankfully—came in a bottle and did not need to be refrigerated.

I paid a token fifty dirhams for the consultation and took a prescription note to the on-site pharmacy. This was a hole in the wall in a basement behind which were utilitarian shelves laden with medicines. There was a not especially long queue ahead of me and, reaching the front of it meant being meted out more of the no-nonsense treatment that I had received in the consultation room.

I went away, having been told to report back in a couple of weeks for a scan and fields tests. I found this a little irritating, as it was not that long since the tests had last been done, but I appreciated that my new carers needed all the information that they could get. Besides, the results had been fine last time, so why be concerned now?

One issue was the cataract. It was still not too noticeable, but, as an English teacher, my job called for a good deal of book-reading, much of it in front of pupils in a classroom situation. It was not lost on me that, in order to see the text, I was having to make the distance between a book and my eyes ever smaller. Apart from this no doubt looking a little odd to the pupils, it could have had classroom management implications: if I was holding a book so close that it prevented my seeing what was going on all around me, all sorts of poor behaviour could have been the result. Things never quite got that bad, but the trend was noticeable.

The classrooms were equipped with screens linked to computers upon which notes, worksheets, PowerPoint presentations and the like could be displayed. It was becoming obvious that I was not able to read everything that the screen might show. To see anything on one, I needed to stand quite close to it and turn towards it—another potential source of poor classroom management.

I made it to the end of the first term. Karen and I celebrated with an Indian meal on the balcony of a restaurant that overlooked the Dubai fountains. We were happy and acted as though our whole lifestyle was blessed. But the truth was that I was unhappy. Not only was I not as enthusiastic about the job as I had hoped to become, but my eye problems were making everything much more difficult than it needed to be. I was doubting the wisdom of returning to school teaching.

After the Christmas break, which was very enjoyable on the whole, I went back to the eye doctor. I had the promised fields test and scan. The former was a challenge. I pretended to myself that the reason was a poor match between my glasses' current prescription and the vision deficiencies for which they were being expected to compensate. The scan was even more disconcerting.

A young female nurse took it. She clearly found photographing my right eye difficult. She took a picture, but it seemed as though it did not show her what she was expecting to see.

'Just a minute,' she said as she adjusted the equipment.

The COVID mask that she was wearing concealed her face, but I had little doubt that it was registering worry. The lines of a frown were visible around her own eyes.

'I just need—'

She exited the room, leaving me with my chin on the rest. A more senior colleague came in to take over. She too was disconcerted by what she could see. Pragmatically, she took a scan anyway and showed me back to the waiting room, where Karen was looking through a magazine. Karen could tell from my face that all was not right.

'What's wrong?' she asked.

'I don't know,' I replied, 'There was a problem with the scan.'

'What sort of problem?'

I shrugged.

I was called back to the consultation room. The bad-tempered doctor was slightly slumped over his desk.

'It's not good news, Adrian,' he told me gravely.

'Oh,' I said, non-plussed.

He put an image on his computer screen. It showed what appeared to be three lines drawn by a child in a row—except that the middle one was some distance below the other two.

'This is your optic nerve,' the doctor explained. 'It is registering minus nine; it should be no more than minus two.'

He declined to say to which eye he was referring. I assumed that it was the troublesome right eye, but I later realised that it must have been the left. I also assumed that this bombshell was the reason for the nurse's problems, but, in the light of later experience, it was probably that she could not see my right optic nerve through the ever-growing cataract. Either way, I was in big trouble. The doctor continued.

'The fields test, too—'

He breathed out dismissively as he threw his hands in the air.

Oh, shit, I thought. This is it. Blindness.

'What can I do?' I asked stoically.

'We'll up the eye drops,' he said, 'There are four drops that you can take. You are currently on three. I will give you a prescription for three medicines—one includes two of the drops. You must take them twice a day. Let's hope that it brings the pressures down so that you can keep the sight that you have got.'

He added ominously.

'Do not ever forget to take the drops.'

I rejoined Karen stunned. We collected the medicines from the on-site pharmacy. That was the beginning of the regime that was to cause me so much angst in that supermarket car park months later.

At work the next day, I told my head of department I was already weighing up the options. I might have to give up the job early. That would not be so bad—it was not one that I was enjoying in any case. But then what? Whatever my accomplishments, that I was going blind was likely to hit my employment prospects.

Even so, I quietly put in a few applications for higher education jobs in the UK. This was not so that I could take advantage of the NHS. To be frank, I did not expect that the care offered back home would trump the private provision that I had become used to abroad. But, if the worst did happen, it would be better that it happened at home, where a support network of family, friends and Tosh would be on hand to supplement Karen's efforts.

I did quite well in terms of securing interviews. Almost all potential employers shortlisted me and, for a few weeks, I was frequently on Microsoft Teams as I tried to sell myself to virtual panels of academics and administrators. In one, the question came up about whether I would be prepared to work overseas. 'Well,' I began in answer, 'speaking from Dubai…'

Offers did not come flooding in, but I was not discouraged. Getting the interviews was a good start and I was confident that one would eventually hit the mark.

While all of this was going on, I found obtaining eye drops to be remarkably easy. They were all available over the counter from any pharmacy. At first, I used the one at Spinneys. Like many supermarkets outside the UK (like the Tesco in Malaysia), Spinneys was not a standalone shop, but the centrepiece of a miniature mall that included other essential outlets, such as banks, hairdressers and somewhere to procure cosmetics and medicines. The café was especially good, too. In order to get my drops, I simply needed to go into the pharmacy and ask for them. The pharmacist would then open a drawer behind the counter, take out the box containing the little bottle and hand it over. It cost about the same as a prescription in the UK.

A few months into our stay, a pharmacy opened in the building in which we lived. It was no longer necessary for me even to go out to pick up the medicine. I had only to take the lift two stories down.

Bad news on jobs continued to come through. I was at the Expo when one rejection email arrived. I checked it on my phone as Karen and I walked towards the exit at which we were going to summon an Uber. We had spent much of that day discussing what to do next in our lives while experiencing the often-bizarre displays that countries from around the world considered represented their cultures. Over a vegan burger at a restaurant inside the Sustainability Pavilion, we considered what a change might bring.

'If I land a job, it will be better for building up my CV than what I am doing,' I assured Karen.

She probed.

'Then what?'

'Who knows?' I shrugged, 'Perhaps go abroad again, but as a

University academic. I think that I need to consider my eyesight. It might be an impediment to anything I do.'

'You'll be all right,' Karen said, with her usual optimism.

She bit into her burger. I was not so sure. The cataract was becoming more noticeable. It was not too debilitating as yet, but it seemed to be progressing with frightening rapidity. I also had to admit, if to no one but myself, that I was excited by the prospect of more change. It was true that we had only been in Dubai for a few months, but it was not offering the hoped-for adventures. This was not to do with the country so much as my circumstances, which were too tied to my job and so not susceptible of the variety that I wanted.

On a February evening in a café in the Mall of the Emirates a new vista finally opened up. I was with Karen and Russ drinking an Americano and nibbling on a macaron when an email flashed on to the front of my phone. It was from Huddersfield University—with whom I had recently had an interview—and it was asking whether I would be available the following day for a conversation.

'That's got to be a job offer,' I said, excitedly.

'You think?' Karen asked.

'Well, what else do they want to talk to me about?' I asked rhetorically, 'To get my predictions for the weekend's footy?'

'Good work, buddy,' Russ said.

He came over as a little disappointed. He had spent years trying to get me to go over to Dubai and now, having turned up, I was leaving again after a not especially lengthy stay. But hopping straight over from Malaysia to the Middle East had probably been a mistake. A bit of time back in the UK between overseas postings would have been sensible. It would have given me the chance to ground myself again. I had not appreciated how weary I was from the four years in Southeast Asia: a little 'battery recharging' had been needed.

Although the meeting with Huddersfield was set up for a specific time, I remained in the flat all day in a state of growing apprehension. It was the half-term holiday, so I did not have work to take my mind off what was about to happen. I am not sure why I did not go out—was I worried that the phone might ring at any moment and I did not want to miss it? When it happened, the offer came through as I had suspected that it would.

It would be wrong to suppose that it was without difficulties. For a start, the job was due to start—really, it had to start—immediately after the Easter break. This meant that I would not be in a position to give the school my contractual notice. Potentially, this had ramifications for my reference, which had not yet been taken up. Indeed, the school was entirely innocent of my job applications. Any negativity that the reference might contain could well have cost me both jobs, the one that I had and the one that I had tentatively been offered.

Equally irksome was the requirement for me to get a medical sign-off from Huddersfield. I remembered the examination before going to Malaysia—again, my fate hung on whether the medical professional to whom I spoke was prepared to ignore my glaucoma.

On this occasion, the chat took the form of a phone call. The nurse who spoke to me asked the standard questions about whether I suffered from anything. Then came the one that I had dreaded: are you on any medications?

'Yes,' I said, 'I take eye drops twice a day. For glaucoma.'

'Mmmm,' she said, 'You might need to have some special software for your computer.'

I assured her that that would not be necessary.

'Okay,' she said, 'I will make a note that you will need an assessment in using IT for possible training.'

I could see no purpose in protesting. The examination was not a bar to my taking up the job, so I resolved to deal with any problems as and when they arose.

After this, there was an interval of a week or two during which references were collected. At the end of it, I was made the formal offer. The school had come through and given me a positive, or at least, fair, reference and all was well.

That really just left nothing to do but the saying goodbye. It was something of a watershed. My adventures abroad were coming to an end—forever? Perhaps. Perhaps not. But, either way, I had a two-year contract with the University that I was determined to see out. For the foreseeable future, I would be swapping the sun and sand of Dubai for the drizzle and cold of the North of England.

A few days before we left, Karen and I met up with Russ at the Dubai Mall for a suitable send-off. We had dinner at our favorite Chinese restaurant and coffee in the shadow of a water feature that consisted of a cascade being surfed by statues of swan diving men apparently attached to the wall by their dicks. My Facebook photographs of the evening were intended to be verité in style, moodily black and white, unposed.

Later, I picked up three months' supply of drops from the pharmacy on the ground floor and packed my bags. After half a decade as a rootless wanderer, I was looking forward to a little stability. In medical terms, I was not to get it.

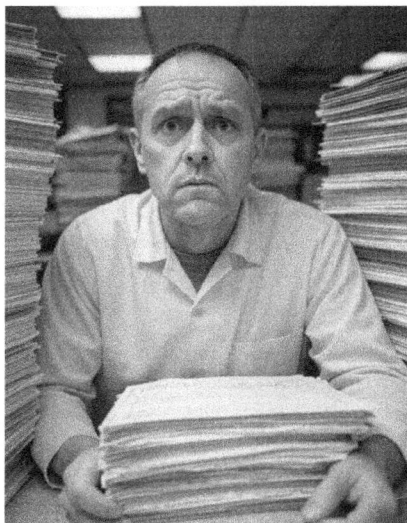

Chapter 14—Long Waits and Dirty Blurs

THE BALL CAME at me with surprising speed and accuracy. It skimmed over the net and hit the ground well within the lines of the serving box.

'Fuck!' I said, rushing forward, stretching out with my racket to scoop it back just before it bounced for a second time.

That kept the rally alive, but it was not anything like a killing blow, the ball meekly landing mid-court and well set up for a baseline smash that would leave me flailing and helpless. Tosh was straight on it, swinging his racket, connecting with force, propelling the ball towards the rear of the court. I scuttled backwards, arcing my racket through a back hand and just about returning it. I followed at a run, seizing control of the net. The ball bounced twice—that was allowed for Tosh—and his arm traced an elegant semi-circle upwards, lobbing me. I could only watch glumly as the ball hit the ground within the baseline before curling into the abyss beyond.

'Jesus!' I cursed, 'I thought that this would be easy! How did you get that good?'

'A bit of practice, mate!' Tosh explained.

'And quite a lot of talent!' I said.

We were playing VI Tennis in a tent in a park on the edge of Nottingham. The game differed from the ordinary version in fewer ways that might be expected. The court was slightly shorter, the ball was slightly larger and it contained a bell so that its position could be ascertained by a person with limited or no vision. Concessions were made to players based on their level of disability. Tosh was classed as B3, which meant that, as I had discovered, he was permitted two bounces. I was in the B5 category, for which no leeway was given—it was one bounce only for me.

It was difficult not to admire Tosh's skill. The rather patronising quarter that I had granted him was dropped: this was going to be a true competition!

He served again. Another good one. I was more prepared this time and sent the ball down the side of the court. He returned it but was now hopelessly out of position. It was child's play to put in a cross-court backhand that won me the point.

'Good shot!' Tosh said.

It would have been fair for him to have spoken with an edge of sarcasm, as if to say, 'well done on exploiting a person's disability', but there was nothing like that in his tone. He was of my mind in wanting this to be a proper contest. Indeed, he went on to hold his serve, his baseline game proving more than a match for my own.

Tosh's serves were underarm, although no less powerful for that. I adopted the more usual overarm style and I could tell that this caused him a few problems at first. He quickly adapted. Several rallies went on for a while, both of us covering plenty of ground. I was at my most successful with drop shots. On several occasions, I was able to dink the ball over the net giving Tosh little chance of reaching it from his preferred station at the back of the court.

We did not play a full match and ended having won an identical number of games. We briefly considered playing a tie-breaker but quite liked the fact that there was no overall winner.

'That was useful,' Tosh said, as we walked off the court, 'It showed me that I need to develop my net game.'

On the next court, a contest was going on between two players, a man and a woman, who were both B1. In other words, they were 'totals'. They were allowed three bounces and played with lowered nets. They were amazingly adept. The man, in particular, being more experienced, played as though he enjoyed perfect vision. Nothing got past him. The woman was newer to the game and sometimes was not too close to the ball as it entered her side of the court. The two had a coach who offered tips and advice. As the ball flew through the air and hit the ground, the bell rang, guiding the players towards it. I suppose that judging where the sound originated was a skill that built up with more and more court time.

The quality of their play could easily have led to condescending claims that they were not disabled, but 'differently abled', or something of the sort. There was, to be sure, something rather wonderful about watching people with no vision whatsoever master, or nearly master, a sport for which vision is usually so central a requirement. But I could not imagine that either of them would not have traded accomplishment at VI Tennis for eyesight. I was reminded of Sharon's session on reading Braille: yes, it was impressive, but that should not detract from the tragedy that is blindness.

For my part, I had enjoyed the game, as both spectator and player. Evidently, so had Tosh, since he expressed a desire for a rematch.

Karen and I were in Nottingham for the weekend, spending time at our main—that is, our own—house. In Huddersfield, we were renting in a town centre complex consisting of an old textile mill that had been redeveloped—isn't everything?—into flats. Its chief virtues were that it was right next to the University and gated, which minimised the danger of unwanted visitors. My commute was to step outside the gate. That was it. That put me on to the campus.

This is a requirement that I have built into my jobs since the time when I had to drive between Wisbech and March just to go to work. When everything is well, commuting is tolerable enough, but, after my bookshop seizure, I was forced to surrender my driving licence for a year and that turned the simple act of being punctual into a living hell. Had it not been for Sally giving me lifts on most days, I would have been stranded. From then on, I always attempted to live within walking distance of work.

Another advantage of the Huddersfield flat was that it was only a few minutes' stroll from the University Health Centre, with which I registered as soon as we moved in. The UK was ahead of Dubai in dropping COVID restrictions. Vaccination clinics, held in various public buildings and branches of Boots, the high street chain pharmacist, were a last vestige of the pandemic that clung on for a few months. They quietly faded away as that whole weird period receded into history. A more serious consequence was the devastation that it had done to the NHS. My failure to get my prescription in Sainsbury's that night would not have happened but for the pandemic.

On which subject, the old familiar clock was ticking. My last appointment in Dubai had been in February. I landed at Birmingham Airport at the end of March. Add on the three or four weeks that it took for my registration at the Health Centre to be completed and I was already approaching the due date for an examination.

I called the Health Centre. This was a strange experience. For a start, it was a couple of minutes before the phone even started to ring in earnest because I was taken through the inevitable message about 'unusually high call volumes' (if the volumes were always high, as they seemed to be, then what was unusual about high call volumes?), then I would finally reach the receptionist who might put me through to a doctor. Fair enough, except that every time I actually went to the Health Centre, it was totally devoid of patients. Listening to those recorded messages, it was easy to believe that it would resemble a field hospital on the Somme, but no! It was a good place to go and get some peace and quiet. On the two occasions that I actually had appointments—neither of which was to do with my eyes—I was seen early by the available medical staff because no one else was around.

Anyway, on that first call I did get through to a doctor. My question was about how to make an appointment to see an eye specialist.

'It could take months,' I was told.

'Really?'

'Yes.'

'But,' I pressed, 'This is quite a serious thing. It's degenerative: the longer this takes, the more I lose. I mean, what eye problems are more serious? Is there no chance of my being prioritised?'

The doctor sighed audibly.

'I could write an email,' she said, 'But I can't promise anything.'

'Thank you,' I said, 'I would appreciate that.'

'If it's just your pressures that you want to get checked,' she advised, 'You could go to Specsavers in town.'

Specsavers was a high street optician, much like the one that had identified my glaucoma in the first place.

'I could,' I replied, somewhat irascibly, 'But I'm not paying taxes to support Specsavers.'

'What can I say?' The doctor said with a roll of the eyes so extreme that I could sense it through the phone, 'It's the best advice that I can give if you want to get some immediate information.'

I went to Specsavers the following weekend. It was a large branch that also offered 'audiology' services—I assumed from this that they had branched out from eyes to ears. It was well-appointed and reminded me of the private medical facilities that I had enjoyed abroad.

'Would I be able to get my eye pressures checked?' I asked the assistant who was acting as de facto receptionist.

'Do you have an appointment?' she asked me.

'No,' I confessed, 'I will make one if I need to, but I am not asking for an eye test. I just want someone to check my pressures and let me know what they are.'

'Wait here,' she said.

She disappeared into the short corridor of consultation rooms behind her. A few minutes later, she returned.

'Would you like to come this way?' she said.

'Oh,' I replied.

This was much more rapid than I had expected. I would have been more than prepared to bag a slot for a quick blast of air on to my eyeballs a week or so later. Yet here I was being shown into a consultation room to be greeted by a green smock-wearing optician.

'You just want me to check your pressures?' he asked.

'Yes. I know that sounds a bit odd, but…'

I went on to explain the problems with getting an NHS appointment.

'Okay.'

I went through the by now second-nature procedure: chin on brace, air squirted into one eye, then the other.

'Right eye, twelve, left, thirteen,' the optician said.

I was delighted. The drops were continuing to work their magic. I was even more delighted when he refused to take payment for the service that he had done me.

I walked out of the shop with Karen, feeling that everything was all right with the world.

But…everything was not all right with the world. I had not really needed the quiet warning that I had been given with that scan in Dubai. The cataract was getting worse. Much worse. And quickly. The vision in my right eye became more and more affected.

It is important to understand what this was like. A cataract is often said to cause the vision to turn milky. This implies that it becomes blurry or something like a 'white out' in a film: annoying, but not incapable of being overcome. It is not like that at all. A cataract is more like a dirtying of the eye's lens. Think of it as being not dissimilar to what happens to a car windscreen in heavy fog. The vision grimes up and darkens, causing everything to look as though it is being seen through filthy dishwater. Colours are flattened out and desaturated. Forms lose their sharpness. By the end, nothing can be seen but blobs of the brighter colours against a charcoal grey background: it is like looking at a Rothko painting in a dark room. When I described this condition to Tosh, he informed me that that was more-or-less what he had been born with and that it had taken fourteen operations in the late 1960s to restore what vision he had. I was sad to hear him talk about how medical science had moved on such that had he been born in, say, 2001, he might well have regained most of his sight.

Over the course of a year or so, my right eye deteriorated badly. In response, my left stepped up. It became stronger. I had already more-

or-less written it off, but, as its companion was increasingly submerged in visual sludge, it shouldered the burden of getting me safely around. This is not to say that it suddenly turned into a digital camera, but—and this sounds bizarre, I know—it saw more. For instance, it had, for years, only been receptive to one line of text at a time. If I closed my right eye and looked at a page in a book, I would see a line of words at the centre of the view, but it would be closed in by smudges of blurred typeface above and below. Not so now. A whole chunk of words was visible. And that was only one way in which my hitherto useless eye proved itself in extremis.

I wondered why this should be so. Aldous Huxley in *The Art of Seeing* writes about the psychological dimensions of sight, of how the operation of the eyes has as much to do with what we believe as what they are physically set up to do. That doctor in March who, all those years ago, dismissed my high pressures, made much the same point: he told me that eyes have a tendency to compensate for each other's deficiencies. He was proving to have been correct.

This should not be overplayed. The world according to my left eye was still a gloomy place, lacking bright colours and filled with many shadowy hollows. But I could at least see it, albeit imperfectly. It was not how I would have wanted to live for long, though. My hope was that a cataract operation lay in my near future. Or my medium-term future. Sometime at any rate.

An appointment for an examination was still not forthcoming. Time passed and I chased my doctor, but she could only reiterate what she had said on the previous occasion: she had informed the local eye hospital. I would just have to wait.

It could have been worse. It was worse for Tosh who was forced to have another emergency operation. The retina in his right eye had aped that of his left and become detached. More silicon oil and more posturing. The oil was removed some months later. The effect on his sight was noticeable – and not in a good way. He reported how, when heading into town—for, as it happened, an operation follow-up—he stepped off the bus and turned to face Nottingham's Market Square, only to be stunned at not being able to see anything because of the glare from the winter sun. It was, he said, the most vulnerable he had ever felt in his life. Photosensitivity had not been a feature of his condition hitherto, but it now presented a major challenge. Sunglasses would not work, as they would simply blackout what little he could see. He eventually found that wearing a baseball cap (either Liverpool FC or Star Trek) helped, but not a lot.

Tosh's biggest grievance was the disruption to his tennis schedule, which had started to occupy more and more of his life. Not only did he train at the weekends, but he was now entering tournaments all around the country, including in Scotland. He attained reasonable levels of success, often making the semi-finals. His *bête noire* was a player who always turned up and who Tosh described as 'playing like he had perfect sight.' He was nigh on unbeatable. Every time Tosh came up against him, Tosh's tournament was over. Psychology probably came in there as with my left eye: Tosh kept on losing because he could not imagine winning.

As the cataract got rapidly thicker and dirtier, I identified ever more closely with the VI community. Mentally, I was preparing for blindness. I knew that my left eye was on the verge of collapse and, even if I had a cataract operation in my right, there was no guarantee that it would improve anything. I could only foresee a future of darkness.

'If I became blind would you leave me?' I asked Karen.

'No,' she replied.

'Would you be willing to be my carer?'

'Yes.'

Her answers were not intended to make me feel better. That was not her style. They were matter-of-fact statements that needed no elaboration. I knew that they carried the truth, or her truth. To me, they offered consolation, but I was feeling bleak and alone.

I was also increasingly concerned for my personal safety. As my vision got worse, my capacity to judge the physical world around me declined. For example, when crossing the road, it is perfectly normal to step out in front of oncoming cars if they are far enough away. Estimating their speed is easy enough and, in any case, drivers can make adjustments in the moment if necessary. I was finding it difficult to be sure how near a car was to me. For all I could tell, it could well have been in a position to knock me down if I ventured into the road. That, of course, is if I saw it at all. More than once, I was about to leave the safety of the pavement only to jump back as some vehicle that I had not seen (often a bicycle) passed me. More generally, I was becoming clumsier and more prone to falling or crashing into things as my sense of three-dimensional space diminished.

I arranged a drink with Tosh, telling him that I needed to 'discuss VI matters'. We met at a pub in Nottingham called The Hop Merchant. We had pencilled in midday, but that was when it opened, so, arriving ten minutes early, I stood on the busy street outside, loitering and brooding. I could read few of the signs on shops, cafes or buses all around me. Crowds were amorphous, like huge crawling creatures moving slowly over the pavement. But my ears were more acute than they had been and I picked up every growling engine, every crying baby, every grumbled 'for fuck's sake'. That, I thought, is one small blessing.

I spotted Tosh. He was carrying a white stick, the device that blind people use to negotiate their way through the world around them. He was walking up from the bus stop on a street that bisected the road in front of me. He could not see me. I wondered what he could see.

'Tosh,' I shouted to gain his attention.

He called back, as chirpy as ever.

'All right, mate?'

'Are you okay?' I asked. I was rather shocked to see the white stick.

'Oh, there's definitely been a deterioration since the operation,' he told me as he reached where I was standing.

Again, I was a little bereft of words.

Tosh's eyesight had been extremely limited beforehand and there had been a deterioration?

'I'm sorry to hear that,' I said, hopelessly.

He just shrugged.

'I've just got to get used to it,' he said.

He told me some of what this now meant for his life. He could only read cooking instructions on food packaging with the aid of his full strength LVAs (Low Vision Aids: very strong readings glasses). Sometimes nothing could help and the small fonts remained invisible to him. If he was alone with Sharon and she needed something to be read, he would either scan it with her phone (an app called Be My Eyes was his recommended method) or photograph it and enlarge the picture. He also struggled with picking up small objects that had fallen to the floor. Sharon often found them before him just by feeling for them.

We made our way into the just-opened pub and bought a couple of drinks. I had a boring lager, Tosh went for a real ale called The Bishop's Wet Fart or something similar. We sat at one of the small tables set up outside with the business of Nottingham as our backdrop and soundtrack.

'What do you want to talk about?' Tosh asked.

I sipped my beer.

What did I want to talk about?

I was not too sure. It was good to be with someone who understood what the world was looking like for me and how I felt about it. Was I treating Tosh like a personal support group? I hoped not, but I could not deny that he did not need to say much in order to be of help. I began by telling him about my ever-variable pressures. He laughed with good-natured irony.

'You're an amateur, mate!' he said, 'Mine have frequently been in the thirties and Kerry—'this was a reference to a member of his VI circle, '—has got pressures in the sixties!'

I was staggered.

'The sixties! I didn't know they could go that high! Her eyes must be about to explode!'

'It's not good!'

'Fucking too right!' I said. 'Makes me feel a bit less bad about my own problems.'

'How bad are things?'

'Pretty bad,' I said, 'My right eye—the one with the cataract—is as good as dead and my left eye has always been shit. I don't know what my percentage of vision is at the moment, but if it's thirty I would be pleased.'

'Fucking hell!'

'Exactly!'

He had a meditative draw on his glass.

'My condition is known as congenital cataracts,' he told me, 'so I know what you're feeling.'

'I suppose,' I went on, 'I am mostly concerned about not being able to read.'

'Ah, well, that's easily solved,' he said, 'Do you use a Kindle?'

'I only ever read on the Kindle app on my phone,' I confirmed, 'It's all that I've been able to see for ages now. Real books are like historical artifacts. Nice to have, but they don't serve much practical purpose anymore.'

This was no exaggeration. It was some time since books had been a comfortable read—as my experience in Dubai had shown.

'Good! Well, increase the size of the font on your Kindle.'

'Can you do that?'

'Yes. What is your current font like?'

I showed him a sample of a book on my phone.

'Jesus!' He said, 'Well, you're going to want the font at least twice that size.'

'I'll give it a go.'

We sat in a meditative silence for a couple of minutes.

'You probably won't go completely blind,' Tosh said at last.

I hoped that he was not erring on the side of the optimistic. It would have been in character for him to do so.

'Probably not,' I said.

I appreciated his help—both verbal and the non-verbal. He had not even been aware of the latter. I nodded and smiled my gratitude, but that was a language which he also could not access. The gestures and facial expressions that are an everyday part of communication in the 'sighted world' are opaque to him. He has likened it to someone sitting in on a conversation in a foreign language that they do not understand. Interestingly, he believes that this particular disability has saved him from many a fight when he has not seen someone giving him 'the evils' across a bar, causing them to walk away in a state of bemusement rather than starting trouble.

I finally got a hospital appointment, but it was not without my having to make a lot of phone calls. I discovered that getting through to anyone in the NHS is about as easy as sending a text message to Julius Caesar. After a good deal of getting nowhere slowly, I found myself talking to a young woman in an office somewhere whose job seemed to be to manage appointments. At first, she told me that I was not on a list for an appointment any time soon. She said that she would double check and she got back to me—she actually called me, which I regarded as a big win—to let me know the date on which I was expected.

The hospital was in the suburbs of Huddersfield. It was—like much of the town—built into a repurposed old industrial building. Inside, however, it was like most such places: somewhat impersonal, bright, emptier of people than seems likely. The eye clinic was on the second floor, which I reached in a lift.

The reception was staffed by a couple of pleasant ladies who met me with big smiles and strong Yorkshire accents. Doctors and nurses wandered around in numbers. I had been nervous but I relaxed upon entering. I was directed to sit in one of the chairs that were set up as a waiting area in the main part of the room. There were not many other patients. Every so often, a nurse, dressed in green scrubs, came in and called a name. In response, someone stood up—sometimes helped by a family member—and followed her or him along a corridor towards a consultation room.

Time passed. My appointment slot came and went.

'I wonder what's happening,' I said to Karen, who sat alongside me.

'I don't know,' she said.

It was odd because the clinic was busy but not exactly overloaded and, as far as I could tell, it was well-run with things happening when they were supposed to.

A nurse came in from the door that led back to the lifts. She held a clipboard.

'Adrian Jarvis?' she called.

I sprang to my feet.

'We were expecting you downstairs,' she told me.

That explained a lot.

'Oh,' I said. 'Is there a bit of the clinic down there?'

'We want to run some tests,' she said, ignoring my question.

On the ground floor, I was taken into a crepuscular room in which were chairs and familiar machines. I was met by a doctor in green scrubs. He took me through the usual menu of pressure tests, scans, fields tests. He did not seem too happy with the results.

'Your pressures are high,' he said.

I was puzzled.

'They were twelve and thirteen when I had them checked in Specsavers,' I said.

'They're nowhere near that now. Nineteen and twenty three.'

The feeling of the ground falling away beneath me to which I had become too accustomed hit again. An emptiness filled me.

'Really?' I said weakly.

'I can't see much of your right optic nerve because of the cataract.'

'I can have an operation on that, can't I?'

He shook his head slightly.

'In theory, but the glaucoma complicates things.'

'It complicates everything.'

'Yes. Glaucoma doesn't have much going for it.'

'What can I do?' I asked.

I was sure that it was not the first time that I had voiced that question.

'I will make an appointment for you to come back in six weeks to see a consultant. Then we can make a decision.'

'Six weeks?'

'Yes,' he said with what appeared to be an air of satisfaction, 'the days when we would say "see you in a year" are over.'

The six weeks passed without my being notified of any appointment. To be fair, the period included the Christmas holiday, during which I let myself forget about medical matters for a few days. But, come the new year, my anxieties returned. I reminded myself of my own words: the longer this takes, the greater my loss. More phone calls. More trying to get through to people.

It was nearly three months before I saw the consultant. She

chastised me about my not leaving a gap between applying different drops, because the eye can only hold one drop of liquid at a time and putting a second one in washes away the first. Perhaps that was why my glaucoma had become so advanced in spite of my devotion to self-medication. Apart from that, she put any decision about longer term treatment off until after the MRI scan.

I didn't get the results of that until I saw a different doctor some weeks later. It was noticeable that appointments suddenly became more frequent. I found that I was not left sitting in the waiting room for too long either.

'The only thing that came back from the MRI scan was that one of the bones in your face contains an unexpected amount of oxygen,' the doctor informed me.

'Is that bad?' I asked.

'I don't know,' she said. 'Probably not or someone would have been in touch. Your face has lots of oxygen in it—everyone's does.'

She took my pressures. They were at an all-time high.

'Twenty six and thirty six,' she said meditatively.

I slumped in my chair.

'Well,' I replied, 'I guess that's it. It is what it is. It's what I've been expecting.'

This was true. I had been mentally preparing for this day for years. Since at least the night of that conversation with David in the bar of the hall of residence in Malaysia. Since my chat with Tosh at the Hop Merchant. Since—well, there had always been a little voice in the back of my head, reminding me of what was coming, like a slave in the chariot of a newly proclaimed Roman emperor.

The doctor looked at me with what can only be called compassion.

'It's not over yet,' she said. 'We can still operate.'

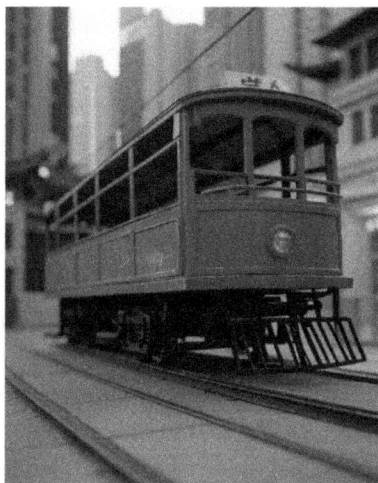

Chapter 15—Postponing the Inevitable

MY MIND WAS not on glaucoma as I sat in the passenger seat of a convertible Bentley speeding over the Oresund Bridge from Denmark into Sweden. The roof was down, the sun was up and ABBA were singing *On and On and On* over the sound system. It was a carefree moment in another road trip with Mike, but it came at a higher cost than it should have done. The holiday had been months in the planning, but now it was upon us, it was cutting across medical arrangements that were still finely balanced and could easily have led to my having to cancel or postpone the treatment that I needed.

That appointment with the doctor in Huddersfield was the point at which my eyes bifurcated, so to speak, and became the responsibility of two different hospitals. She ended by telling me that she was going to refer me to the glaucoma department at the hospital in the city of Leeds. This was not too much of a hardship—Huddersfield to Leeds is a brisk seventeen minutes by train—but it seemed that it was only going to apply to my left eye. My right eye was still going to be dealt with in Huddersfield. This was a function of the cataract. I could have that operated on where I was, but the more advanced surgery required by my left eye needed specialists from elsewhere.

Hearteningly, the difficulties around the cataract surgery that had been hinted at by other doctors were no longer referenced. It seemed that it would be a relatively straightforward operation and I could expect it to be successful. I was also going to have at least one iStent installed. This was often done at the same time as cataract surgery. It was less radical than whatever the Leeds people would do but was still aimed at relieving the glaucoma.

An iStent is a minute valve that is inserted into the eye's drainage channels to help relieve pressure. The doctor gave me an iPad with an explanatory video on it, although that consisted of a soundless animation which did little to illustrate exactly what would happen. I was just happy to learn that the cataract would be fixed and at least some of my vision would return. I gladly signed the proffered release form. From then on, it was just a case of waiting to be called for the surgery.

My first appointment in Leeds followed soon after. Since she happened to be free, Karen took me in the car. I had given up driving many months earlier. Upon our return from Dubai, we had bought ourselves a rubbish hatchback—the days of MX5s and MR2s were behind me for now—and had shared the driving.

This worked well enough until I began to realise that my vision was simply not up to it and that I was risking not only our lives, but those of any poor unfortunates who I might fail to spot and run over. I made my decision to stop when I went to collect Karen from a leisure centre in which she had been teaching yoga. It was after dark and I could see nothing through the windscreen apart from an impressionist painting of colour from cars' headlamps, cars' brake lamps and the street lighting overhead. Everything was a splash of brightness in which nothing assumed a definite form. The road was invisible and pedestrians were ghosts.

As we pulled into the car park of the Seacroft Hospital in Leeds, I was hit with a sense of very English mundanity. I had visited eye doctors at slick modern complexes in Kuala Lumpur and Dubai, but this was a rather old-fashioned low-rise brick pile at the end of a drive surrounded by lawns and trees. It could have been a school from the 1940s—which was somehow therapeutic in itself. Through the modest wooden door, we found ourselves in a long, narrow corridor with signs showing us the way to the various departments. The eye clinic was highlighted in yellow. The corridors were, a wall display helpfully explained, a relic of the hospital's past as a centre for the treatment of infectious diseases. The belief was that creating as much distance as possible between wards would prevent cross contamination. I have no reason to suppose that this did not work, but, in the present, it made for a lengthy stroll before anything like a doctor or nurse could be found. There was no one else around. I have often mused on how dangerous hospitals might be—in theory. Anyone could have walked into those corridors at will and were they minded to do harm to whoever they bumped into, it would have been quite some time before help could arrive.

The corridor reached an end, turned right, passed a small café area that was closed (I would go on to discover that it almost always was) carried on for a while, turned left and finally led me to a door into a waiting room. Behind a low desk sat a woman in a nurse's uniform.

'Hello,' I said to her, 'I have an appointment.'

'Name and date of birth?' she demanded.

I supplied the information and was told to take a seat. The seats were not fixed and some had been moved together, presumably by couples or groups, a practice that was obviously tolerated. There were few other people there. I passed the time by checking Facebook. A post advertised a book by Paul McCartney. A radio that was on at low volume in the room's background was playing, *Got My Mind Set On You* by George Harrison. A patient walked in and, when asked for his name, gave 'John Lemon'. It occurred to me that I had paid for our parking using the RingGo app. I hoped that by the end of the afternoon, no one would be able to say to me You Won't See Me. As for my glaucoma, I certainly did not want to Let It Be.

A nurse came to the waiting room door and called my name. I got up and was led across a corridor to a consultation room. She tested my vision—pretty hopeless—and took my pressures—off the charts—and returned me to the waiting room.

The time for my appointment was receding into a distant past when I was finally called through by a very tall surgeon. He had fair skin and freckles—much like my own. He examined my eyes, giving special attention to the left. He asked a colleague from another room to join him. This guy was around my height and owned a good full head of hair. He had a quick look at my eyes. The two of them shared a few half-muttered phrases of the type, 'See?' And 'Yes..' and 'Mmm, yes..'

'Laser treatment would not do any good,' the tall surgeon said at last.

I already suspected as much.

'We can operate,' he continued.

'That is where you jab a hole in my eyeball?' I asked.

'Yes, a trabeculectomy,' his shorter colleague said.

'There is a small chance of it not working,' the tall surgeon said, 'but it should stabilise things.'

'You probably wouldn't need to use eye drops any more either,' his colleague added.

'But I'm addicted!' I burst out, 'What would I do without having eye drops to look forward to?'

This was only partly a joke. I do not suppose that it is possible to become addicted to the drops in any literal sense, but I certainly spent quite a lot of the average day in anticipation of the moment when I would apply them. Quite apart from the good that I hoped that it was doing for me, the few minutes in which the soothing wash of liquid slooshed over the smooth surface of my eyeballs were always an oasis of private relief in a wilderness of stress from work, relationships or whatever. The need to continue moistening my eyes with artificial tears was not much compensation for its loss.

'Would you be prepared to have the operation?' the tall surgeon asked me.

'Yes,' I said.

Yes! Yes! It was what I wanted more than anything.

I knew that it would not end my problems—nothing could do that—but just to achieve some sort of resolution... that would be—well, beyond a dream, really.

'Do you want a local or general anaesthetic?'

'I'm in your hands.'

The two doctors exchanged a glance.

'We would usually go for local,' the tall surgeon said.

'Local it is,' I said.

Tosh always favoured general, since he had no desire to be conscious while his eyeballs were being prodded and poked. In any case, part of his condition was something called *nystagmus*, which was involuntary movements of the eyes: it would have been dangerous for him to be awake while a surgeon was attempting to cut into eyes that were not still.

I signed another release form and returned to my life, longing for the call to come summoning me to the operation. I was now on two waiting lists.

In the car on the way back to Huddersfield, I thought about what I was letting myself in for. There was an urgency about the doctors that only confirmed how much of an emergency case I, or at any rate, my left eye, had become. The heady days when the doctor in Malaysia sent me away with a few reassuring words felt like an eternity ago. I could hardly believe the rapidity with which I had reached where I now was.

Then there was the small matter of needles. Both of the operations for which I was scheduled would involve needles being inserted into my eyes. That, I feel safe in saying, is one of the most horrid images any of us can conceive. It is simply not a nice thing to think about! But here I was, willingly allowing myself to undergo it. I pushed the thought into that section of my mind labelled, 'deal with it when you come to it.'

Scheduling the operation proved to be more of a problem than it should have been. The tall surgeon was going to be doing it, but it was the summer and everyone—including me—had holiday booked. My commitment to that road trip in July was long-standing and the surgeon was due to take some leave almost as soon as I returned to the country. The operation was pushed back to October. The same fate befell the cataract operation, but that was hit with two blockages. The road trip was one, but, on top of that, I had to travel to Hong Kong in early September to teach. Frantic phone calls resulted in a decision: I would have the operation the day after I landed back at Manchester Airport. It all made for a rather pressured start to the Autumn Term.

Vile Jelly

So it was that I arrived at the Eurostar Flexi-Lounge in Folkestone at the start of the road trip feeling like I was on my last break before something momentous was going to happen. It was the evening and therefore not busy. Apart from the bored staff, Mike and I were the only ones in there. We stocked up on coffee, snacks and sandwiches ahead of taking the Bentley on to the train for the crossing. We had already discussed what we would do upon disembarking. Visits to museums and other places of interest were top of the list. It was going to be a journey for which a keen pair of eyes would be a benefit—it's called 'sightseeing' for a reason.

Interestingly, Tosh informed me that VI people, even totals, use the same word, despite its being meaningless to them. Indeed, as he asked, what do blind people actually get out of travel? He mentioned some of his total friends who would profess a love for a certain place and would talk about its unique characteristics, irrespective of how minimal their sense of its uniqueness must have been.

An experience that does not need much vision is hurtling through the night in a powerful open-topped car. That is a sensation beyond sight. I cannot say why it is so special. But, when I drove sports cars of my own, I always relished the summer darkness when I could fold back the roof and confront the universe on its own ever-mobile terms. The sensation of having nothing above but infinite space: that is real freedom. On that first day of the road trip, we arrived in Calais at around ten o'clock with a three-hour drive to our first hotel which was located on the edge of Bruges in Belgium.

After a night of fitful sleep, we headed north. It was another long day of motoring; we were meeting Eddie, a friend of ours from University, in Hamburg that evening. The temperature was high. That whole summer was hot—probably the hottest on record, since they're all the hottest on record these days. I had bought myself a little trilby from a golf shop in Dubai and it served to keep the sun off what Mike had charitably described as my 'slap head'. I wore my jacket to keep my arms from burning and stored the eye drops in one of its pockets. This was so that they would be readily available when I needed to take them. Having taken the consultant's advice to revert to a system of spacing out the applications, I took the drops over the course of an hour; this would likely fall while we were on the road. Occasionally, I reached into the pocket to ensure that the drops were still there, although there was nowhere that they could have gone for as long as I was in the passenger seat of the car. The tips of my fingers connected with plastic bottles that were hot—too hot, I worried.

We reached the hotel close to Hamburg Airport well before the drops needed to be put in. Eddie met us in the bar and we all took a taxi to a restaurant on the edge of the park in the Winterhude area of the city. We sat at a table on the edge of a lake. The shores were edged with the deep greens of deciduous trees. The surface of the water was a pattern of rich blues. Nearby, white masts thrust upwards from boats moored at a marina. Here and there, raised sails were pale wedges against the cloudless sky. It was a dream of European life—a visual dream.

Our conversation dwelt on medical matters. That was standard these days. The only people who seemed to think that I was in any way young were my eye doctors—they constantly harped on about how glaucoma as advanced as mine was more common in people who were older than me, much older! My eyes were only one of many ailments discussed that evening. Both Mike and Eddie had had health scares that had necessitated their undergoing extensive checks. Neither had tested positive for anything. My own recent 'MOT' blood test had shown that I was pretty fit—apart from my eyes. But the demonic spectre of bodily decay lurked in the mysterious realm to which we were all heading on tickets that were strictly one way.

The next morning, Mike and I set off for Sweden. We were going to pass all the way through Denmark in one epic drive. The German autobahns gave us the opportunity to get some miles on the clock. The car's speed rarely dropped below a hundred miles per hour; at our fastest, we touched a hundred and sixty.

In Stockholm, I munched on reindeer and lingonberries with a growing unease. At the Vasa Museum, I strolled around the salvaged remains of a wrecked wooden battleship, not seeing the details. Our guide pointed out carved figures on the rotund sides of the hulk: I could only make out their broad shapes. The armour, or weaponry, or headwear that he was describing were obscure to me. On a boat tour around the harbour, I could not read the signs on buildings, or make out the tracery on windows, or identify the shrubbery in gardens.

Again, Tosh had a useful opinion about this. In speaking of a trip he had taken to Marrakech, he mentioned how he picked up some visual details, or listened to descriptions from sighted friends or tour guides but also concentrated on what his other senses were telling him. He could certainly see some of the vibrant colours of the souks, or the brightness of the clothes and jewellery on sale, or the displaying cobras of the snake charmers who set up their stalls in the squares, but, more vividly, he heard the sound montage of a busy African market, the calls of sellers, the enthusiastic acceptances or polite—and not so polite— refusals of prospective buyers, the increasingly high-pitched roar of accelerating motorbikes. Then there were the smells—of spice, mint tea, roses and shit. Perhaps this was one answer to his own question about what VI people get from travel. Another came from a holiday he took to Rome on which he rejected a visit to the Vatican on the grounds that Sharon did not want to take part in an experience that they had been warned was almost exclusively visual and therefore of little value to them.

By the time Mike and I made it back to Copenhagen, I was ready for an operation, but I still had one more journey to make before that could happen. As, a couple of months later, I sat on the plane from Manchester to Dubai for the first leg of my flight to Hong Kong, it struck me that the cataract was now about as bad as it could get. My right eye was to all intents and purposes blind. Smudges of muddy colour were all I could see through it. I willed it to be otherwise, but psychology can only get you so far. I watched films and TV shows on the in-flight entertainment, seeing less than I should have done. By now, faces had ceased to be contoured; noses had been replaced with blurs; eyes were generic holes. In Dubai Airport, I used the interval between flights to catch up on my emails. I sat in a café, booting up my University laptop. I could only make out anything on the screen by getting so close to it that I could feel its heat on my skin. Arriving in Hong Kong, I took a taxi in the dark to my hotel. Outside of its windows was the now constant Jackson Pollock painting of artificial lights. The city was a black smudge.

My lessons took place at a teaching centre in the Wan Chai district. It was a well-appointed and very efficiently run place. The faces of my ten students were undifferentiated discs. The screen upon which my PowerPoint slides were displayed was a square of blank light. I needed to stand directly in front of it to see anything at all. Fortunately, I was fully conversant with the module by this stage and could teach it with only passing reference to the slides.

I taught on two consecutive weekends—all day on both Saturday and Sunday. Because of this, I could claw back some leisure time on the weekdays in between. I took the opportunity to explore. I was reminded of the craziness of Hong Kong, a different type of craziness from that of any other city. The streets crowded and noisy. The roads locked up with cars, buses, lorries. The old-fashioned trams quaint and toylike in the midst of so much modernity. The contrasts: cheap cafes and snack bars right next to grand malls and skyscrapers with names like 'Virtue Building'. The sizzle of oil in woks, the insistent note of sounded horns, the incessant babble of voices. It was a workout for all five senses. The certainties of the West rubbing up against the constant negotiations of the East. I was reminded of Tosh's descriptions of Marrakech.

Back at the hotel in the evenings, I fell into a habit of having a drink—a coffee for the most part—in the bar that occupied a portion of the lobby. A door led to an exterior terrace. As such places go, it was not too distinguished: more a smoking deck than a place to luxuriate. It included a few comfortable chairs and low tables, on each of which was an ashtray that was overflowing regardless of the hour.

I sat out there, with a car park and road in front of me, closing my eyes in turn, searching for a way to convince myself that I could live like this. I never succeeded. But, more hopefully, the operation was coming that could make a difference: it might be life-changing.

As my stay wore on, the reality of what I was about to undergo became more and more my one thought.

Was I afraid?

No. It was not fear as such. It was more a sense of being on one side of a ravine, needing to be on the other side and being aware that there was nothing in between but danger, however survivable, however minimal. I had been told repeatedly that the chances of failure were vanishingly low, but there was a chance: someone had to be the unlucky one.

Why not me? What made me special?

If I could have projected myself through the next few days, I would have done so. I focused intently on how I would feel once they were over. In my imagination, I created that place of the future and pretended that I was already in it.

The tactic worked for a while.

But as I touched down in Manchester on a Monday at midday, I could only think of what I would be going through on Tuesday...

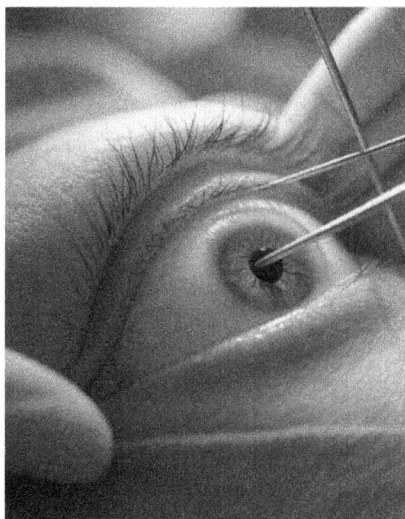

Chapter 16—Needles in my Eyes

STRANGE CANDY COLOURS. Amoeba shapes moving in front of me. A dark background. Muddy. I could see nothing else. But, all around, I could hear calm voices. Blades, they said. Washes. Can you pass me the...

I was ready for it. I knew from the pre-op appointments. One at each hospital.

The whir of something.

A drill?

Maybe.

The pre-op nurses had asked: do you suffer from any of the following? No, I said. What about this? Not that. No again. They had said, let me just check the...

Cool water splashed on my eyeball. My lids pinned back and useless.

You're fine, the pre-op nurses had said. You can go ahead with the operation.

Now there I lay on a gurney. A mask on my face covered everything apart from my right eye.

Vile Jelly

I had arrived in that room in the most banal way possible—by waking up, getting dressed and setting off as though heading out to do some shopping. I had been told to report to the hospital, which was in the nearby town of Halifax, at seven o'clock in the morning, with the proviso that I could be waiting for several hours before the operation took place. Karen drove me. We didn't talk much on the way. My silence was nerves, hers simple concentration.

I had some idea of what to expect. A few weeks earlier, my Mum, by pure coincidence, had had a cataract removed and replaced with an artificial lens. She was reporting complete success—so much so, indeed, that the surgeon was suggesting that she be used as a model of how well these things can go. I felt a strange resentment at that. I was yet to be given my appointment at that point and in conversations with Karen, I railed at my retired mother being given the treatment, while I, who was still economically active, languished on a waiting list.

Of course, in part, this was because of constraints that I had myself imposed. I was off travelling and not available. I realised even as I spoke that I was being unfair, but I was expressing a deeper worry.

What if my operation was not as successful as Mum's? What if it were altogether a failure?

I felt that it would be my failure, that I would be in some obscure way inadequate. I was—I accept—being irrational, but strange things go through your mind when you are shortly to have needles poked into your eyes.

In the hospital, I was directed to the surgical ward, an unexpectedly ordinary place. There was a pre-op area, which only patients were permitted to enter, although a nurse, spotting Karen and other partners sitting alone in the corridor, allowed them in. So, Karen was alongside me as I was prepared for what was to come.

The space consisted of comfortable chairs arranged in a horseshoe pattern, each with a low table alongside it. A nurse appeared and asked me some questions and gave me a few physical checks. It was effectively the pre-op examination again. I suppose that they had to be sure that I was fit for what was to come. To my delight, my blood pressure was about perfect and my resting heart rate low. Another check later confirmed that this had been no fluke.

Sitting opposite was a guy around my age who was scheduled to go in before me. He wore an expression of stoic acceptance. I imagined that I did, too. He answered the questions that the nurse put to him desultorily. I didn't hear what he was there for, but it was a safe bet that his affliction was similar to mine. An older woman was there because her glaucoma had started to give her pains around the face and forehead. A guy who looked ancient was there for cataracts. We conversed, like— I would say soldiers about to go into battle, but it turned out that he had actually been a soldier. And, from what he said, he was well-travelled. I did not ask whether he had ever been in action, but his eyes must have seen many things that mine would not have wanted to see. The guy around my age was an odd job man. His condition was affecting his capacity to take on work. It was a reminder that eye diseases have serious economic consequences for their sufferers.

I learned that I was third in the queue for the operation. This meant that I would be in that room for a while. I was glad that Karen was there. We talked idly about the future. It was an apt topic since it seemed that it might be better than we had feared. If, of course, the operation were a success...

I was finally taken through to the operating theatre. There was no smock, no requirement for me to take off my shoes. I simply lay on a gurney and was wheeled in. The mask was applied. I could not really tell who else was in the room, but it was clearly several people. My right eye was rubbed with a numbing solution. The anaesthetic? No. That came with the first needle.

I had been told that the eye does not feel pain. Even without the initial rub, the needle would not have hurt. Perhaps that is true. I did not feel pain, certainly, but I was conscious that a needle was being pushed through the delicate shell of my cornea. It was not a comfortable sensation. Neither was it as terrifying as it could have been. The surgeons all around me treated it as nothing out of the ordinary. What effect the anesthetic had on my vision, I could not say: the eye was pretty much blind in any case.

The operation began. For around forty minutes, I watched a 1970s art film as the weird blobs moved in front of me. That was the cataract operation completed. Now it was time for the iStent.

'Would you like to do this?' a man's voice said.

'Yes,' a woman replied.

I recognised the voice. It was the doctor, the surgeon, who had been treating me.

More needles. I felt them more clearly. Was the anaesthetic wearing off? It may have been that this stage of the operation was simply more needle-heavy. I heard the sound of a spring. I was not sure what it meant, but I guessed that it was a device that was moving the iStent into place. One iStent went in without problems. The surgeon prepared the second. I heard the spring...

'Stop moving!' the surgeon said sharply.

'Sorry,' I said.

I was not sure that I had moved, but she went on.

'Even a small movement—a tiny movement—can cause this not to work.'

Another woman's voice spoke up.

'Has that one not gone in?'

'I am not sure,' said the surgeon.

'I think it's there on the eyeball,' the other woman said.

'Wash it away with some fluid,' the man said.

I felt cool water on my eye.

'I'll try another one,' the surgeon said.

I heard the springing noise and felt the unyielding metal of the needle in my eye.

'Has it gone in?' the other woman asked.

'I can't tell,' the surgeon said.

'One is definitely in,' the man said.

'Leave it at that,' the other woman said.

Suddenly, the mask was removed.

'You can sit up,' the man said.

I swung my legs to the side of the table.

I could see nothing out of my right eye. Only blackness. It was worse than the cataract had been. At least with that, I could make out some colours, however weakly. Now: nothing. Through my left eye, I could see that the voices belonged to my regular doctor, who had been the iStent surgeon, a male doctor of around my age and a woman also around my age. With them were a few assistants. I mentioned that I could not see anything.

'I know it's disappointing,' the man said. 'But give it time.'

One of the assistants put a plastic patch over my eye. It was transparent, but the tape that held it in place blocked most of the view— or would have done, if I had had any. It was to prevent me from scratching—which was the worst thing I could do.

I returned to the pre-op area and took the seat next to Karen's. The odd job man was also out of surgery and sat opposite with a patch of his own. He was subdued and concentrated.

'Everything okay?' Karen asked.

'I think so,' I replied.

To be honest, I was not sure.

A nurse made us both a coffee and offered us biscuits. Through the tape I was beginning to see something like the world as it had been during the worst days of the cataract. It was an improvement on the immediate aftermath of the operation, but not on how things had been before it.

I was discharged and we went back to Huddersfield. I was given some steroid and antibiotic drops that I had to put into my right eye every four hours—on top of the glaucoma drops and the artificial tears. I was not unhappy about what I had just been through, but I was realistic about it. I was beginning to accept that it would not make much difference to my eyesight.

But, that evening, something fabulous happened. I was sitting on the sofa in the flat and I happened to glance over towards the kitchen area. Through the tapes I could see—well, I could see. And not just see. There was a clarity and sharpness to everything, to the uprights of the dining table legs, to the curves of the kettle, to the red LED numbers on the front of the microwave. It was all still obscured by the patch, but the darkness, the gloom, had gone away.

The next morning, I removed the patch to discover that the vision in my right eye was better than it had ever been. Even at its best in the past, there had always been a slight haziness, a flattening out of distances, a mild sfumato effect. That had gone, to be replaced with precision. And the colours! Was the world really that bright? I stared at my phone: the screen was electric with light. The Facebook app was not the deep royal blue that I had been seeing, but a vivid and attention-grabbing ultramarine. It was as though my eye had been upgraded from analogue to digital. Best of all: it was no longer short-sighted. My left still was, it must be said, but it ceded its crown to the right; it was again the servant. The right eye was master. For the first time since the age of twelve, I could operate in the world without the aid of glasses. There was a side of me that wanted to weep for the geeky kid that I had been when those boring plastic frames first entered my life; he had, apparently, only ever been a simple operation away from perfect sight!

I experimented with my new-found vision and quickly found that it was not perfect after all. I had been warned that, although my long-distance vision would be excellent, the same would not be the case with my near vision. I found that I could now read the number plates of cars on faraway roads but put a page directly in front of my face and it was a blur. Oh well! I was more than willing to take that for the prospect of not having to wear glasses full time again!

There was also the matter of the dots. I could see deep black blotches floating in front of me, like full stops or flicked ink. I worried that this might mean that the operation had not worked. After all, my eye had been cut open—who knows what could have got in there! I Googled 'black dots after cataract surgery'. The ever-soothing internet assured me that the effect was natural and would pass. I was only a little mollified. For some reason, I decided not to mention the dots to anyone, least of all my doctor, as though to do so would be to invite them to stay forever.

I had an appointment at Huddersfield eye hospital the day after the operation. I drove myself there. Drove! And exited the lift to the clinic with a spring in my step. I announced myself to the receptionist and ensconced myself in a chair in the waiting area like a character in a musical, my movements light and choreographed, a contrast to the hunched shoulders and air of resignation that I had brought with me on my last visit.

The doctor herself collected me from the reception.

As we walked to her office, she said: 'You seem to be jolly.'

'Yes,' I said gleefully, 'and you will notice that I am not wearing glasses.'

The pressure in my right eye was down, although it was not as low as I would have liked. I didn't care. One iStent had attached itself. Two would have been ideal, but the doctor was happy and reassured me that there was nothing to be too concerned about.

'It's good to see how upbeat you are,' she concluded, 'you were very despondent last time.'

'This is the best gift I have ever been given,' I told her, 'I have worn glasses since I was a kid. To be able to live without them is—I don't know what to say. It's incredible.'

It was the best of times, but I was only halfway through the ordeal of operations. I still had the trabeculectomy on my left eye to come. My appointment was set for about a week later. It was to be at St James University Hospital in Leeds. This was the place at which a terrorist who had planned to blow up as many nurses as possible had been talked down by a patient taking a break. As a medical facility, it was a step up in scale from Seacroft. As Karen drove me towards the relevant ward, it was like passing through a small town. Halls of residence for nursing students rose up on either side of us. Departments for various ailments were not a couple of rooms in a larger building, but hangar-size edifices in their own right.

We parked and headed into the reception area. It was, again, about seven in the morning so there was no one around and nothing was open. I needed to go to the toilet. Appallingly, I walked into the Gents to see an old toothless guy squatting in a urinal having a shit. This, he told me, was because the one cubicle was occupied and he was unable to 'hold it in any longer'. I decided that I could wait. Were I superstitious, I might have seen that as a bad omen.

In the ward, I was escorted into the patients' waiting room. It was almost identical to the one in Halifax, comfortable chairs in a horseshoe shape with a small square table alongside each. This time, Karen was obliged to stay outside. I called her on my phone to suggest that she go somewhere and come back later. She said that she might, but, typically, she didn't: she stayed to support me, if only from a chilly corridor.

Again, I was some way down the waiting list. I could do nothing but sit, reading on my phone—at least as well as my new lens would permit. When I was finally called, it was into an anteroom to the operating theatre. I lay on a gurney with the anesthetist and her assistant looming over me.

'Oh, wow!' the assistant said. 'You've got lovely eyelashes!'

'Everyone says that,' I replied, 'I think that they are the one bit of me that is actually beautiful. Everything else looks like Shrek after he's decided to stop trying and really let himself go, but my eyelashes— they're knockout.'

'Well, I need to just get through your beautiful eyelashes to your eye,' said the anesthetist drily. She rubbed my eye with the numbing substance. The cold steel of a needle flashed in front of me. As in Halifax, it didn't hurt, but I was aware of it entering my eyeball. It stayed there for some time. I could feel my eye bulge: was it being filled with some new substance? Did it have the room for that?

The anesthetist checked her handiwork. She seemed satisfied. After a few minutes, I was wheeled into the operating theatre.

This time, I was physically lower than I had been in Halifax. Somewhere over my head, I could hear the voice of the tall surgeon. The phantom figures of others moved around in the room's unseeable spaces.

'Can you stay still for about forty-five minutes?' the surgeon asked.

'Yes,' I said.

I was terrified of moving at all after what had happened in Halifax. Losing an iStent was one thing, but this time my eye could end up sliced in two. I lay still with my feet slightly apart and my arms by my side.

My eye was stabbed and jabbed. Again, this was accompanied by a calm professional soundtrack of the medical personnel talking. I had no idea what was happening.

About halfway through, the surgeon asked me: 'Everything all right?'

'Yes,' I joked, 'It's like being at a spa. Quite relaxing, to be honest.'

This was true. I was feeling unaccountably sleepy. I supposed that falling unconscious would probably have not been a great idea.

'You're doing really well,' the surgeon assured me.

The operation continued. I felt no pain. The anesthetist had done a good job.

'Nearly finished,' the surgeon said.

'Oh,' I said, surprised. It had all happened much more quickly than I had expected it to. The obligatory patch was attached to my face and I was wheeled out.

I returned to the waiting room and had my tea and biscuits. Other recent operands were sitting around. I was discharged with an appointment set for the next day.

I soon had to come back. The prescription that I had been given to take to the hospital's pharmacy was unsigned. I returned to the ward to find that the tall surgeon had already left for home. A bit of hanging around later, a different doctor had lent their monogram and I grabbed my latest collection of drops.

There was not to be the same revelation as with the first operation. I had anticipated that. In some respects, I was bound to experience a letdown. After all, nothing was being improved this time. At best, I could only anticipate things remaining as they were. That was not really what would happen.

On the plus side, the black dots disappeared.

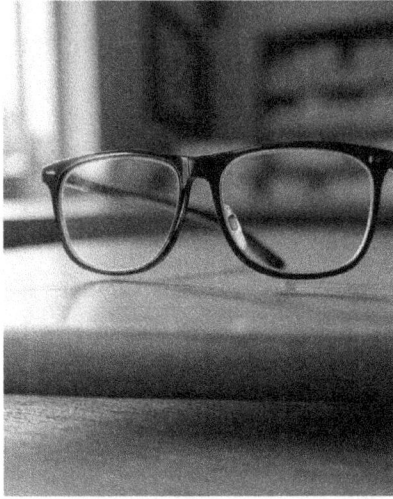

Chapter 17—Post-Op

'NINETEEN,' THE TALL surgeon said.

I was in his office twenty-four hours after the trabeculectomy having the pressure in my left eye taken. It was lower than it had been, but higher than I had hoped for. The surgeon pondered for a few seconds.

'I'll take out a stitch,' he said, 'I can guarantee that that will bring down the pressure.'

'I've got a stitch?' I asked.

'Two,' he said, 'I'll take out one now. We might take out the other next week.'

He produced a device that was essentially a pair of tweezers and told me to look down. I did so and felt a mild pricking in my eye.

'Ow!' I said.

'Sorry!' the surgeon said.

The stitch gone, he gave my eyeball a gentle squeeze and took the pressure again.

'Thirteen,' he said.

'That was a quick change!' I said, impressed.

He chuckled.

'Yes, pressures go up and down all the time. You're mostly doing okay. I will see you next week.'

I left the hospital and took an Uber to Leeds railway station. I was on my own this time since Karen was away working in Lincolnshire. I had a coffee in the fast health food restaurant Pret a Manger, experimentally closing my right eye to test the vision in my left. It was not too good. I had been assured that it would take somewhere around six weeks for the eye to finally settle and that I could expect it to be sub-optimal for much of that time. I could only imagine that any improvement would have to be substantial for it to get back to anywhere near where it had been. The world as seen by it now was blurry and granular. Not only were edges not crisp and sharp, but most objects did not appear to have edges at all. I completely lost a lot of things that, as confirmed by my right eye, were prominent in their spaces.

On top of that, I was banned from taking strenuous exercise or even bending over. This would not be forever, of course. Even so, it threatened to drastically affect my fitness and was a problem to someone who insisted on shoelaces. I often mistakenly broke this rule. I would bend over in the kitchen to retrieve a dropped object or would pick up some socks from the bedroom floor. There would follow a period of my worrying that I had rendered both operations void and would wake up the next morning stone blind.

More positively, I was expressly forbidden from putting any drops in my left eye apart from the steroids and, when needed, artificial tears. Once the steroid course was over, there would, all being well, be no requirement for me to put glaucoma drops into my left eye, perhaps for the rest of my life. It would still be afflicted, but, as far as I would be concerned, it would be normal, just doing what eyes are meant to do. It all promised to be excellent news. Provided that my vision returned.

For a while, I became something of a human pinball, bouncing between follow-up appointments in Huddersfield for my right eye and in Leeds for my left. On one occasion, I had appointments in both places on the same day—Huddersfield in the morning, Leeds in the afternoon. It was difficult to keep track of them all. I found myself constantly checking my calendar to make sure that I was not inadvertently missing one.

At my second Leeds appointment, I discovered that my left-eye pressure had dropped to sixteen. This was progress, but the possibility that my pressures might be too low—a danger of the operation—did not look like it was going to happen. The second stitch came out at that point. Now it was up to my eye to form a bubble over the hole that had been prodded in it so that the surplus aqueous humour could drain away unnoticed. I was assured that things were largely going according to plan.

I had no reason to doubt it, but I could not avoid the dawning realisation that the vision in my left eye was not going to recover fully. To some extent I could attribute this to psychological factors: as my right eye grew stronger, my left relaxed back to its life of unapologetic underachievement. But it was delusional to suppose that physical factors did not also come into play.

I tried putting on my glasses. What they revealed was not the—albeit indistinct but—discernible reality that had been mine while the cataract did its worst. Now, it was only a slight improvement on the view without glasses. Short sighted and then some. I reasoned that I could get a stronger lens prescription. But it would not make that much difference. I was reminded of the words of that consultant in Huddersfield who had warned that interventions would not be without risk. She had been right. Unfortunately, the risk had not paid off. Or, at least, it had not paid off as well as it might have done.

I had missed a couple of my teaching periods at the University to have the operations. I did not take any further time off, opting to return to work the following day. This was to the amazement of the nurses at the hospitals, who counseled a period of rest, but, as I pointed out, I spent a lot of time at work writing on a computer—which was exactly what I would have done during a period of convalescence. Ergo, I might as well go back to work.

I was touched by the concern of my students for my wellbeing. Most were from abroad—various African countries, Pakistan, Sri Lanka, sometimes India. A couple of guys from Nigeria were particularly keen to ensure that I was all right.

'How are your eyes, sir?' one asked.

'They're okay,' I replied. 'Recovering.'

He was genuinely pleased.

'But you should be resting,' he went on.

'What?' I said. 'And miss being with you guys? No chance!'

In fact, teaching suddenly took on whole new dimensions. As in Hong Kong, I used a large screen at the front of the class and, as in Hong Kong, this had been causing me difficulties for a while. No longer! I could stand at the back of the classroom and get a sharp, perfect view of whatever was being displayed. I had frankly forgotten how black text on a screen could be. For so long, it had appeared to me grey and fuzzy. I had accepted this and assumed that it was just printed that way. I had to adjust to seeing it as it was intended to be seen.

But teaching was fun again! I could give up trying to conceal my lack of vision. And I had been doing that. Instead, I could now stand at the huge sweeping window of the teaching room taking in the vista of the town stretching out below me and seeing everything. I could read both the prices on the sign for the petrol station opposite and the number plates of cars parked in submissive rows in the car park next to it—the very same car park in which I had nearly panicked at the unavailability of my eye drops all those months earlier. I could follow the monumental white curves of the football stadium's supporting structures peeping up over the buildings and trees in the middle distance.

None of that, however, completely compensated for the undeniable fact that my near vision was atrocious. Holding a book, my phone, the label of an eye drop bottle, up close to my unaided eyes revealed only the sloshing waters of blur. Reading the screen of my computer at work could only be done if I sat some distance from it and enlarged whatever document I was working with to a minimum of one hundred and fifty percent of its default size. I could only see anything on the screen of my iPad if I put my face embarrassingly close to it.

During one of my visits to Leeds, I had my vision checked without the help of glasses, which I had forgotten to take. Right eye? I could read the bottom line of text without a problem. Left eye? Nothing. Not even the top letter, which was around the size of a small elephant. Even standing closer to the chart did not improve matters. The 'top letter in the room' of my conversation with the surgeon was that the operation on my left eye had not been a complete success. It had brought down the pressure and obviated the need for me to take drops, but at what cost? Both eyes together were enjoying a less than happy working relationship.

I would need to find some solution if life were to be tolerable. If there was one place I did not foresee it originating, it was my mother, yet, she was, indeed, its unwitting provider. She was still recovering from her own cataract operations and was suffering from much the same problems as myself. I called her one morning from Costa Coffee in the town's main shopping centre, Kingsgate: I often wondered why almost every mall in England was something-gate, Queensgate, Westgate, Eastgate, whatever. Were any of them built on the sites of the gates of long-gone city walls? The café was one that I particularly liked because it was not enclosed but part of the concourse, giving it it a busy, sociable, air. I sat in a large wing backed armchair and called.

'Hello?' Mum answered.

She sounded as though she had no clue who it could be, despite my regularly calling at that time.

'It's me,' I said.

'Oh, hello Me,' she said.

'How are you?' I asked.

'Okay,' she replied, 'but I'm fed up with my eyesight.'

This was an odd statement given how well her operations had gone.

'What's wrong with it?'

'I just can't read anything.'

This sounded very familiar.

'Neither can I. It's pretty awful. I'm looking forward to getting some new lenses for my glasses, but the doctor has told me not to waste my money until my eyes have settled down.'

'Mine did, too,' she said. 'He told me that I should buy a cheap pair from Boots or somewhere.'

'Can you do that?' I asked, puzzled, 'Wouldn't you need a prescription?'

'You can buy reading glasses for about a fiver,' she said, 'I keep meaning to give it a go.'

I was dismissive of the idea.

'I think that I need to get proper lenses in my frames.'

'Probably eventually, but you should seek out the Boots glasses. Give it a go. You never know—it might work out well.'

For the moment, that was that.

Some better news from my most recent appointment was that I could go back to taking exercise. I celebrated by accompanying Karen to yoga. This had been a longstanding shared activity for us that had been interrupted by Malaysia and COVID. We always did it at a studio in Nottingham located in an unprepossessing industrial estate. It was an unlikely haven of calm and peace. The wooden floor was polished, the lighting was muted and the single window was covered by a thick curtain, lending a cosiness that was totally appropriate to the main activity that the place hosted. Around a dozen participants assembled and lined up on either side of the room, facing towards the centre.

The session began with us all moving to the edges of our mats and raising our praying hands towards the ceiling. We bent over and the movement about which I had been most apprehensive arrived. The downward dog. My hands found the ground on either side of my feet. I stepped backwards, first my right leg, then my left. I raised my buttocks. My head was now upside down. Not only was it facing the ground but held in that position. I waited for the instructor to move us on to the next exercise. On his command, I flowed into lying on my front. I could sense no ill effects. It was all fine. I had no headache. My vision was unaffected. Amid the audible breathing of my fellow yoga practitioners, I let out a quiet sigh of relief.

Work, on the other hand, was becoming difficult again. That I was at that moment writing and editing two research articles only added to my misery. I am sure that a massive stylistic howler that got through with one of them was because I simply couldn't make out the words clearly enough on the screen to notice that I had used the same rather glib phrase twice in the same paragraph—the second paragraph of the whole piece, as it happened. I was distraught when it was published still bearing the error.

'I'm not sure what to do,' I said to Karen one evening as we sat in the local branch of Caffé Nero.

She cradled her hot chocolate.

'You could try getting some cheap glasses like your mum said,' she suggested.

I put down my Americano.

'I have never seen things like that on sale,' I said, 'I'm not sure what she's talking about.'

'Why don't we have a look?' Karen said.

'I suppose I could,' I agreed.

We finished our drinks and strolled down to Boots, which was no more than a few metres away. Inside, I decided to start my search in the same area that carried the false tears that I habitually bought—for a teeth-itchingly high price—when my prescription ones ran down and I had not ordered any replacements.

To my surprise, there was a small section labelled, Reading Glasses. Various frames, mostly of the unfashionable variety, hung from pegs with lenses installed. I picked one up. It had a cardboard backing on which a lens strength was written, in this instance -3. In a state of some bemusement, I removed the glasses and put them on.

In its own, small, way it was as life-changing a moment as removing the eye patch after my cataract operation had been. I was stunned by the clarity it brought. I held up the front of my iPhone. I had been used to having to put it within millimeters of my face, but, suddenly, it was as sharp as Zorro's blade. I had to hold it some distance away to get the best focus—a normal distance away. I was utterly, completely, but pleasantly, flabbergasted.

'How much are these?' I asked no-one in particular.

I checked the price. Ten pounds. Ten pounds for such a transformation! It was impossible to believe. Were miracles really so cheap? I took the glasses off and peered again at the phone's screen. It was back to what it had been. It was worse than it had been. My eyes had seemingly enjoyed looking through the glasses so much that they had no desire to ever go back! They were making their feelings felt in the most robust of ways! I put the glasses back on. Yes, the improvement was frankly remarkable.

I paid the ten pounds and carried the glasses home as though damaging them would be worse than murder. They had to be treated with care. They could not, under any circumstances, be broken.

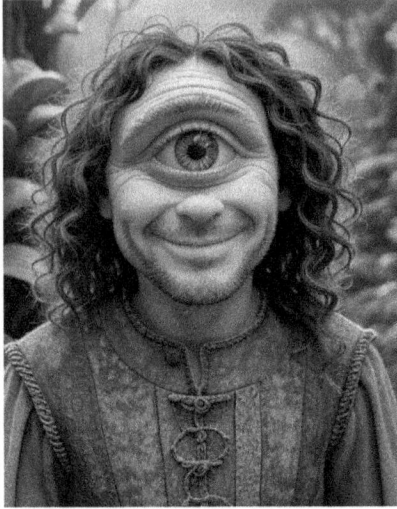

Epilogue—Land of the Blind

I MET TOSH at the Hop Merchant. He arrived with his white stick.

He greeted me.

'All right, mate?'

'Yes, mate,' I returned, 'Shall we go in?'

It was January. I was still enjoying some time off from work after Christmas. Nottingham was cold; the freezing breath that hung in front of our faces was like dry ice from some cheesy 1970s musical. We quickly found a table inside. I ordered a boring lager. Tosh had a real ale called The Drayman's Hairy Arse or something similar.

The previous day, I had attended my last follow-up appointment in Leeds. From then on, I would revert to a more usual pattern of appointments. The news had generally been good. I had taken my glasses—not the cheap Boots pair, but the ones that I had been using for years. As a result, my left eye vision test was not quite as appalling as it had been, although, admittedly, it was still not overly reassuring. My right eye, the test for which, again, I took unaided, elicited from the surgeon the comment that its vision was 'amazing'. It followed the outcomes from a fields test that I had taken in Huddersfield a couple of weeks earlier that had revealed no meaningful loss in my right eye. As I had long suspected, the culprit there had not been my eye so much as the lenses that I was using to boost it. The surgeon took my pressures: thirteen in my right, sixteen in my left. In other words, fine.

It was thus that I met Tosh in a generally positive mood. His operations, too, were behind him. He was moving forward. His pressures were also down. We were, as we settled into that old fashioned English pub with its bar pumps and battered wooden tables and stained-glass windows, both in a good place.

Of course, we were still hostages to our eyes and always would be. My right might have been 'amazing', but it was glaucomatous and needed careful monitoring. It had to be doused with chemicals twice a day. Yes, the iStent meant that I was now on two drops a day, rather than three, but there was no guarantee that the eye would always be so co-operative. Its pressure could go shooting up again without warning and then what? I would be back to three drops a day? Or would I be booked in for an operation to put in another iStent? Both were possibilities. At the back of everything was the knowledge that my optic nerve could collapse and then no lens in the world would be of use. I would just have to hope that AI, or some other technological breakthrough, would come to the rescue.

As for my left eye, it was nice to not have to put drops into it, but the surgeon had warned that if the pressures went up and stayed up, it might be necessary to return to a partial regime of medication. It was a little disheartening to hear, but that eye had been so ravaged by years of disease that the struggle to save it was very real. Perhaps the operation had not yielded the optimum result, but what if it had not been done at all? The urgency with which the various medical practitioners had moved once they got a sense of how bad the situation had become spoke for itself.

I could not pretend that it was not pretty desperate.

On that note, a tribute should be paid to Britain's National Health Service, the NHS. Once occupying the status of secular religion, it had recently lost much of its standing. The pandemic had not been good for it. Initially celebrated—the lockdown had seen the rise of a practice called 'clapping for carers' which called for members of the public to stand on their doorsteps on Thursday evenings applauding—it was subject to increasing criticism as the crisis wore on. TikTok videos of nurses doing undeniably choreographed dances while on night shifts were not considered to be quite as charming as their creators intended: the question, 'why are they farting about with this when they should be treating COVID victims' was often asked. The vaccines that the NHS pushed were also attacked, either as useless, or dangerous—although the latter was more the province of conspiracy theory. The service that the NHS provided was hit badly by the strain on resources entailed by the pandemic and its aftermath, although they could not be blamed for that. Friends had been scathing of the organisation and some had given up on it altogether, taking out private policies to cover their needs.

None of that seemed very fair from my perspective. I had received private care in Malaysia and Dubai that had been excellent. But in retrospect, those doctors had been more concerned with managing my situation than improving it. They had primed me to expect the operations and had first alerted me to the seriousness of my glaucoma, but they had neither taken nor proposed much in the way of practical action.

Only the doctors and surgeons back in the UK had concertedly roused themselves in my cause. On returning from abroad, I had been kept waiting for quite a while, that was true, but, from the second that I had finally entered the system, I could not offer one complaint about the care that I had been given. It is probably not too much to say that the NHS saved my sight. It is definitely not too much to say that it improved the quality of my life.

I will sort out some proper glasses in the near future. For now, the Boots pair are doing a superb job. Using my iPad—as I am while typing these words—has become a pleasure once more. I can even read proper print books again. To be sure, the glasses do nothing for my left eye, but they add to the superhuman qualities of my right and my combined vision is still better than it has ever been before.

I had been using my phone's Kindle app as I had been waiting for Tosh.

As we sipped our beers, he got the conversation going by asking:
'So how are things?'
'Really good!' I replied.
'Nice one!' he said.

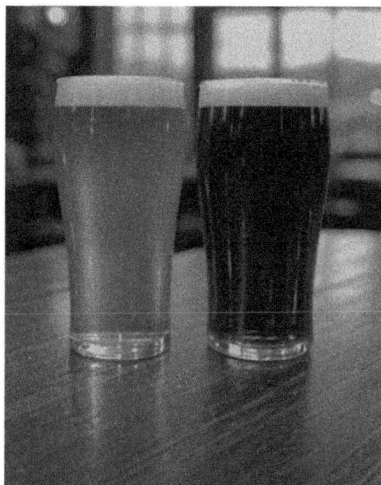